Discharge Planning
for the Elderly

Kimberly Dash, MPH, is a curriculum developer and project director with the Center for Health Care Practice at Education Development Center (EDC) in Newton, Massachusetts. Over the past 7 years, she has been involved in the design and evaluation of several projects related to improving or enhancing public health and clinical content in nursing education and practice: developing an educational program for school nurses to increase their role in comprehensive school health; evaluating "Choose Nursing in the Nineties," a program designed to recruit and prepare minority high-school students for careers in nursing; disseminating six nursing practice models to improve clinical nursing care for elderly patients; preparing teaching materials for nursing, medical, and public health faculty on the science of injury prevention; training nurses from a variety of settings to provide appropriate assessment, management, and outreach to high-risk perinatal clients; and designing educational materials to help nurses better understand the distinction between delirium and dementia, recognize behaviors seen in each condition, and implement appropriate nursing interventions.

Nancy C. Zarle, RN, MS, is director of the Wellness Center and Assistant Professor of Nursing at Aurora University, Aurora, Illinois. Prior to that she was the continuing care nurse specialist at Beth Israel Hospital in Boston, MA, heading a comprehensive discharge planning program for elderly patients and producing a variety of strategies and tools for effective continuing care management. While at the Beth Israel Hospital, Ms. Zarle also served as the principal investigator for the original "Discharge Planning for the Elderly" program.

Lydia O'Donnell, EdD, is a senior scientist and director of the Center for Health Care Practice at EDC. Over the past 8 years she has led a number of research and demonstration projects in the areas of aging, women's health, and community-based prevention services. As part of this work, she has examined multidisciplinary team approaches to health care delivery and, in particular, how nurses can be prepared to assume leadership roles in clinic, hospital, home-based, and community services.

Cheryl Vince-Whitman, EdM, is senior vice president at EDC, and director of EDC's Health and Human Development Programs (HHD). HHD's mission is to promote health, prevent disease, and create safe environments for people of all ages by strengthening the capacity of systems (health care, education, and criminal justice) that affect the lives of millions of people. Trained in psychology, education, and business, Ms. Vince-Whitman has held a leading role in advancing EDC's work in the field of nursing education, research, and practice.

Discharge Planning for the Elderly

A Guide For Nurses

Kimberly Dash, MPH
Nancy C. Zarle, RN, MS
Lydia O'Donnell, EdD
Cheryl Vince-Whitman, EdM

SPRINGER PUBLISHING COMPANY

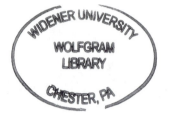
Copyright © 1996 by Springer Publishing Company, Inc.

Springer Publishing Company, Inc.
536 Broadway
New York, NY 10012-3955

Cover design by Tom Yabut
Production Editor: Pam Lankas

96 97 98 99 00 / 5 4 3 2 1

Library of Congress Cataloging-in-Publication Data

Discharge planning for the elderly: a guide for nurses /
   Kimberly Dash . . . [et al.], editors.
     p. cm.
   Includes bibliographical references and index.
   ISBN 0-8261-9230-0
   1. Geriatric nursing. 2. Hospitals—Admission and discharge.
3. Hospitals—Aftercare. 4. Nurse and patient. 5. Aged—Medical
care. I. Dash, Kimberly.
   [DNLM: 1. Patient Discharge—programmed instruction.
2. Patient Discharge—nurses' instruction. 3. Continuity of Patient
Care—programmed instruction. 4. Continuity of Patient
Care—nurses' instruction. WX 18.2 D611 1996]
RC954.D55 1996
362.1'9897—dc20
DNLM/DLC
for Library of Congress   95-25626
                                                   CIP

Printed in the United States of America

CONTENTS

ACKNOWLEDGMENTS

Discharge Planning for the Elderly was originally developed by staff at Education Development Center, Inc. (EDC) and the Beth Israel Hospital (BIH) in Boston, Massachusetts, as a continuing education curriculum for nurses in New England hospitals. Curriculum development involved the active and intense collaboration of many individuals. The authors are indebted to each of them.

We acknowledge the guidance and support provided by the Division of Nursing, Bureau of Health Professions, Health Resources and Services Administration, Department of Health and Human Services. In particular, our project officer, Elaine Cohen, MS, RN, was helpful and responsive to the development of the program, providing feedback and input at various stages of the process.

A group of five advisory board members provided technical assistance throughout the development process. These individuals brought to the project diverse and extensive experience in nursing practice and education, gerontology, and discharge planning. They included: Terry Fulmer, RN, PhD, Professor and Associate Dean for Research, Columbia University School of Nursing; Linda Kaeser, RN, MSW, PhD, Director, University of Texas Health Science Center Interdisciplinary Center on Aging and the Associate Director of the Texas Consortium of Geriatric Education Centers; Linda Redford, RN, PhD, Regional Director to the National Council on Aging's Institute on Community-Based Long Term Care; May Wykle, PhD, RN, Florence Cellar Professor, Associate Dean, and Director of the University Center on Aging, Frances Payne Bolton School of Nursing, Case Western Reserve University; and Carolyn Waltz, PhD, Professor and Coordinator of Evaluation, University of Maryland School of Nursing.

Joyce Clifford, RN, MSN, BIH Vice President of Nursing and Nurse in Chief, and Eileen Hodgman, RN, MSN, BIH Center for the Advancement in Nursing Practice, provided early guidance in curriculum content and design.

In addition, BIH faculty members were instrumental in developing and teaching the original sessions of the discharge planning curriculum. These faculty included: Susan Burns-Tisdale, BSN, MPH; Ellen Kitchen, RN, MS; Jane Matlaw, LICSW, ACSW; Nancy Miller, RN, MS; Marion Phipps, RN, MS; Catherine Reilly-Morency, BSN, MS; Veronica Rempusheski, MS, PhD; and Bonnie Jean Teitleman, MSW. In addition to these faculty, EDC consultants, Jeanne Lowenthal, RN, and Anne Glickman, EdM, CAS, and EDC Staff, Cynthia Lang, provided crucial input into the development of the original program.

We would also like to extend a special thanks to Amy Miller for her assistance in pulling together the original version of this program and to the following individuals for their assistance and support in preparing the educational program for publication: Philip McGaw, Heidi LaFleche, Harriet Dishman, Jennifer Roscoe, Michele Caterina, Jeanine Merrigan, Christopher Hass, and Jennifer Davis-Kay.

PREFACE

The Division of Nursing, Bureau of Health Professions, Health Resources and Services Administration contracted with EDC and the Beth Israel Hospital to develop *Discharge Planning for the Elderly*, an intensive continuing education program for the acute care or bedside nurse. This book is based on this program. The educational program was designed to address the impact of the Prospective Payment System and it's associated diagnostic-related groups (DRGs) on the nature of hospital stays for elderly individuals and to help nurses meet the new challenges associated with this policy change. Specifically, it aimed to improve the quality of services delivered to the increasing number of frail elderly being discharged sicker and quicker from acute care settings. The reason behind this focus on nurses was the growing realization that clinical nurses who provide direct care are in an ideal situation to assess elderly patients' needs and develop continuing care plans that ease their transition from the hospital to home and community.

Ideally, continuing care is the coordination of services to patients prior to hospitalization, during hospitalization, and following hospitalization. As part of continuing care, discharge planning is the process that matches patients' health care needs with available resources at home, in the hospital, and in the community. Careful discharge planning is necessary for high-quality patient care and sound patient management practices.

Traditionally, the responsibility for discharge planning has rested with social service departments rather than nurses. Social workers have played and will continue to play a key role in evaluating the emotional and environmental needs, the strengths, limitations, coping capacity, and resources available to patients and their families. Yet the increasing number of frail elderly patients demands an interdisciplinary approach to the problems and issues of continuing care. This book emphasizes the importance of the interdisciplinary process and recognizes that when physicians, nurses, patients, and their families also get involved, the process of discharge planning is far more comprehensive and even more likely to ensure appropriate continuing care. Specifically, this book elucidates the roles nurses can play as vital members of the interdisciplinary continuing care team.

Preparing nurses for expanded roles in continuing care is essential. Evidence shows that involving nurses in the process of discharge planning makes a difference in the quality of geriatric health care. A recent study demonstrated that comprehensive discharge planning designed for the elderly and implemented by nurse specialists not only improved patient outcomes after hospital discharge, but also demonstrated the potential for reducing care costs by delaying or preventing rehospitalization (Naylor et al., 1994). Yet, despite the effectiveness of comprehensive nurse-lead discharge planning programs, many nurses do not feel adequately prepared to assume new responsibilities in discharge planning. Indeed, one study noted that while most nurses acknowledged the importance of nursing leadership in providing continuity of care throughout the discharge planning process, few understood how discharge planning was accomplished in their hospital and believed orientation was not adequate (Lowenstein & Hoff, 1994).

The need for information on discharge planning is great at nursing undergraduate, graduate, and continuing education levels. Despite the call for nurses to get involved in continuing care, few have had any formal training in continuing care and discharge planning. There are currently no clinical specialist tracks that focus on discharge planning; the topic when covered in nursing school is scattered through the curricula with no solid focus on the fundamentals of gerontology and discharge planning. Similarly, there are few comprehensive continuing education programs for practicing nurses who want to increase their skills in this area in response to their patients' needs. As a result, today's practicing nurses may not be prepared in this area and new graduate nurses come to the hospital setting with varying amounts of preparation in this field.

Discharge Planning for the Elderly was designed to fill this gap in nursing education. With the charge from the Division of Nursing, EDC and BIH developed, implemented, and evaluated an educational program to ensure that nurse participants gain knowledge and skills in (a) applying the nursing process in the practice of continuing care, (b) gerontological nursing, (c) clinical and functional assessment of the elderly patient, and (d) matching appropriate services and resources in the community to patient needs.

This program not only prepares nurses to be more actively involved in the discharge planning and continuing care process, but also to change and improve that process and thus, ultimately, to improve patient outcomes. We do not prescribe how nurses should become more involved in discharge planning at their institutions, but rather provide a variety of options. The book recognizes that nurses' roles in the discharge planning process may vary from institution to institution, as will the models of discharge planning or continuing care in place. However, we address the basic problem-solving skills that nurses need to become more involved in discharge planning and serve as a vital resource to their nursing departments.

PHILOSOPHY OF THE PROGRAM

Advisory board members, EDC staff, and BIH faculty met early in the program development process to outline the training program. As part of that meeting, the staff, faculty, and advisors agreed that the program should highlight the following basic nursing skills:

- Patient, caregiver, community, home, and nursing home assessment
- Communication with the patient and with the continuing care team
- Goal setting and problem solving for institutional change
- Patient advocacy

A major premise of the program and of this book is that nurses should be involved in the discharge planning process from the first day of the patient's hospitalization. Nursing skills should be used to assess patients' needs and prepare them for returning to the community, thus assuring that the elderly receive the services they require once they have been discharged from the acute care setting. Throughout the book, we stress the need for multidisciplinary coordination and communication with others involved in discharge planning, including physicians, social workers, and designated discharge planners.

The chapters provide nurses with opportunities to improve their abilities to assess patients' physical, mental, and functional needs and match patient needs with appropriate resources in the home, community, or institutional setting. The book helps nurses understand that discharge planning occurs in the context of what elders need and want, and what services in the hospital, at home, and in the community, they can turn to for help. Nurses following the program through this book consider the hierarchy of needs, including food, shelter, and support, and what independence and dependence means for the elderly, both able and disabled. The program promotes the philosophy that nurses are patient advocates on both an individual and policy level. As such they should be able to communicate well with their clients and be aware of the current state of gerontological services, both locally and nationally.

GOALS OF THE PROGRAM

The overall goals of the program are to:

- Expand nurses' roles in discharge planning in order to improve the continuing care delivered to elderly patients in the hospital, home, and community
- Improve nurses' skills in assessment of the physical, mental, and functional health status of elderly patients
- Improve nurses' ability to communicate with the elderly and their loved ones in order to ascertain patients' wishes, resources, and needs
- Assist nurses in the identification and evaluation of resources available to the elderly beyond the acute care setting, including family, friends, neighbors, and community-based services
- Involve nurses in the development and evaluation of discharge plans and procedures
- Strengthen nurses' roles in delivering patient education to ensure that patients have the knowledge, skills, and resources to meet their continuing care needs after discharge
- Improve nurses' abilities to address patients' needs along the complete wellness–illness continuum, including the needs of the dying patient

- Help nurses define realistic roles in discharge planning, set personal career goals, and increase their satisfaction with and commitment to geriatric care
- Improve discharge planning at the nurses' home institutions by more effectively matching the patients being discharged with available community resources

REFERENCES

Lowenstein, A. J., & Hoff, P. S. (1994). Discharge planning: A study of nursing staff involvement. *Journal of Nursing Administration, 24,* 45–50.

Naylor, M., Brooten, D., Jones, R., Lavizzo-Mourey, R., Mezey, M., & Pauly, M. (1994). Comprehensive discharge planning for the hospitalized elderly. *Annals of Internal Medicine, 120,* 999–1006.

Chapter 1

WHY IS DISCHARGE PLANNING CRITICAL TODAY?

LEARNING OBJECTIVES

At the end of the chapter, readers will be able to:

1. Describe the health status of older people in America
2. Identify and balance the elderly's needs for independence and dependence
3. Provide an overview of formal and informal resources available to the elderly
4. Recognize critical health care dilemmas confronting health professionals and the elderly
5. Describe the impact of economic realities on the provision of services
6. Outline the philosophy and objectives of continuing care and the process and practice of discharge planning
7. Define nurses' roles in discharge planning

With the introduction of the Prospective Payment System (PPS), the nature of hospital stays has changed dramatically. As a result, nurses today face new challenges in providing continuing care to the elderly. One of the most prevalent ethical issues they face is how to balance their concerns for discharging sick elderly people too soon with the institutional constraints of cost containment (Fulmer, Ashley, & Reilly, 1986). Nurses on the unit have expressed their fears about sending patients home with ill-defined or inappropriate services.

1

This chapter provides readers with an overview of health care issues facing today's older Americans, hospitalization as a critical event in the lives of elderly people, and how effective continuing care and discharge planning can meet their specific needs.

The chapter opens with a discussion of the critical issues affecting discharge planning for the elderly. It then reviews a brief case and, based on that case, describes how to construct a web chart to aid in developing discharge plans that address not only older persons' needs for continuing care provided by others, but also their need to maintain independence and autonomy. The web chart is followed by a true/false quiz that gives you a chance to assess your own understanding of the health care needs and resources of the elderly. A more detailed discussion of discharge issues and procedures follow the quiz.

CRITICAL ISSUES IN DISCHARGE PLANNING

A variety of critical issues influence the discharge planning process. Issues are likely to fall into the following categories:

- Communication (e.g., communication among health care providers, patient/provider communication, communication with diverse groups of elderly)
- Assessment (e.g., patient's perception of health)
- Ethical issues (e.g., preserving patient autonomy while balancing patient needs of dependence and independence)
- Economic trends (e.g., increasing cost of health care)
- Regulatory environment (e.g., the Prospective Payment System and diagnostic-related groups)
- Patient outcomes (e.g., poor effects of hospitalization on the elderly)
- Institutional environment (e.g., hospital administration's receptivity to new discharge-planning protocols)
- Caregiver issues (e.g., increasing numbers of patients cared for in the home, balancing needs of the patient with the needs of the caregiver)
- Community resources (e.g., availability of community services for the elderly, access to services)

- Evaluating and rewriting discharge plans (e.g., protocols for patient follow-up)

The Discharge Needs and Resources of One Patient

The web chart is a strategy that enables one to view a lot of varied information about a patient. The web chart allows one to think about and view the social, economic, clinical, and environmental factors that affect patients and enables nurses to think about those factors as they consider the continuing care needs of older individuals. Second, web charting addresses the nurses' ability to look not only at older people's needs for continuing care provided by others, but also at their need and right to maintain independence and autonomy. Focused on meeting patients' care needs, health professionals and family members often overlook or devalue older individuals' rights to make decisions on their own behalf. Through this exercise, nurses begin thinking about what role they can take, as members of a discharge planning team, to protect the patients' rights to make decisions about their care at the same time that they are addressing the patients' need to accept ongoing help from others.

The following is an individual case study, from which you can construct a web chart to better understand the issues involved.

Case Study: *Mrs. Ruiz*

Mrs. Ruiz, a 75-year-old Spanish-speaking woman who speaks no English, has breast cancer. She lives alone in a two-family home, close to nieces and nephews who all have young children. Her only income comes from the apartment she rents out. She does not drive and relies on buses and relatives for transportation.

Mrs. Ruiz has a previous history of hypertension managed with medication. Relatives report recent changes in mentation, forgetfulness, in particular.

Mrs. Ruiz is hospitalized for breast cancer and has a modified radical mastectomy followed by a good recovery. She still has the dressing in place, which requires daily changes.

The treatment plan is to begin chemotherapy as an outpatient in the oncology clinic located at the hospital.

What information should be considered in developing a discharge plan. Write the patient's name in the center of a blank page and circle it.

Build a "web" of information around the patient's name. Put more generic information close to the patient's name, and link related ideas by lines. Your web may develop something like the example pictured in Figure 1.1.

Questions to Consider

1. What does the chart tell you about Mrs. Ruiz?

2. What factors do you think are particularly important to consider in planning Mrs. Ruiz's continuing care?

3. What are Mrs. Ruiz's dependency needs?

4. What factors express Mrs. Ruiz's need and capacity for independence?

5. What ideas do you have for Mrs. Ruiz's discharge plans that would support her autonomy and also meet her need for support systems?

6. What do you think nurses can do, as members of a discharge planning team, to find an appropriate balance between older patients' independence and dependency needs?

When older persons require ongoing care it is very easy for health professionals and family members to become so caught up in addressing care needs that they overlook the fact that the patients themselves are capable of making many of the decisions about their continuing care. Autonomy—the need to have control over one's own life—is a fundamental need, and loss of that control can adversely affect health. In their review of the literature on aging, Drs. Rowe and Kahn (1987) found much evidence to support the notion that older people who depend on others become happier, more active, and healthier when the degree of control they have over their daily lives increases. A more recent study suggests that the right balance of dependence and independence may vary for different patients.

BEGINNING OF ACTIVITY

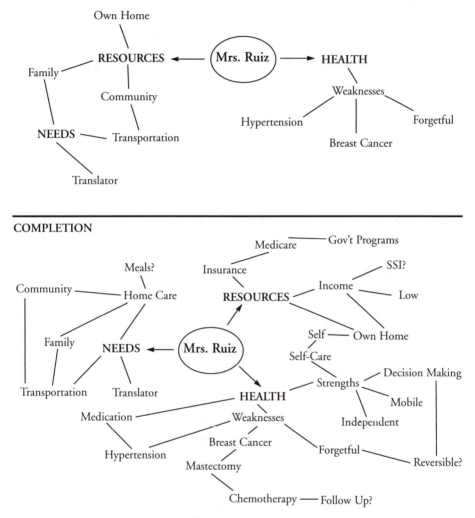

FIGURE 1.1   Construction of a web chart.

Elderly patients with a strong internal locus of control are more likely than those with low expectations for internal control to experience psychological postdischarge distress when they perceive lack of control around their discharge plan decisions (Coulton, Dunkle, Hang, Chow, & Vielhaber, 1989). In their discharge planning role, nurses are in a position to guard and facilitate patients' rights to participate in decisions about their care and to work together to help patients find the right balance between dependency and independence. As advocates for their patients, nurses need to be aware of the factors that may limit patient control, such as speaking with families about the discharge plan separate from the patient (Coulton et al., 1989).

WHO ARE THE ELDERLY IN THE UNITED STATES?

Take a quick quiz. This quiz is for your own information only; it is not a test. Rather, this quiz is designed to stimulate thinking about common myths and facts about aging. Answers are at the back of the chapter, in Appendix A.

The Facts on Aging Quiz

Please circle T (true) or F (false) for each question.

1. People between the ages of 65 and 85 constitute the fastest growing age group in the United States.   T   F   Don't Know

2. Health care costs for the elderly are increasing at the same rate that the elderly population itself is increasing.   T   F   Don't Know

3. Almost half of all the money spent on health care for the elderly is for inpatient care in short-stay hospitals   T   F   Don't Know

4. Among the elderly who require long-term care services, the vast majority live in the community rather than nursing homes or other long-term care facilities.   T   F   Don't Know

5. Most people become senile if they live long enough.   T   F   Don't Know

6. Alzheimer's disease (progressive senile dementia) is the most common type of chronic cognitive impairment among the aged.   T   F   Don't Know

7. Many of the disabilities of the elderly that used to be associated with the aging process are now understood to be the direct effects of illness.   T   F   Don't Know

8. A person's height tends to decline in old age.   T   F   Don't Know

9. More older persons (65 or over) have chronic illnesses that limit their activity than do younger persons.   T   F   Don't Know

10. Older persons have more acute (short-term) illnesses than do younger persons.   T   F   Don't Know

11. Older persons have more injuries in the home than younger persons.   T   F   Don't Know

12. Older workers have less absenteeism than do younger workers.   T   F   Don't Know

13. Blacks' life expectancy at age 65 is about the same as whites'.   T   F   Don't Know

14. Men's life expectancy at age 65 is about the same as women's.   T   F   Don't Know

15. Medicare pays over half of the medical expenses for the aged.   T   F   Don't Know

16. Social Security benefits automatically increase with inflation.   T   F   Don't Know

17. Supplemental Security Income guarantees a minimum income for needy aged.   T   F   Don't Know

18. The aged do not get their proportionate share of the nation's income.   T   F   Don't Know

19. The aged have higher rates of criminal victimization than younger persons.   T   F   Don't Know

20. The aged are more fearful of crime than are younger persons.   T   F   Don't Know

21. The aged are the most law abiding of all adult age groups.   T   F   Don't Know

22. There are about equal numbers of widows and widowers among the aged.   T   F   Don't Know

23. More of the aged vote than any other age group.   T   F   Don't Know

24. There are proportionately more older persons in public office than in the total population.   T   F   Don't Know

25. The proportion of blacks among the aged is growing.   T   F   Don't Know

26. Participation in voluntary organizations (churches and clubs) tends to decline among the healthy aged.   T   F   Don't Know

27. The majority of old people live alone.   T   F   Don't Know

28. The aged have a lower rate of poverty than the rest of the population.   T   F   Don't Know

29. The rate of poverty among aged blacks is about three times as high as among aged whites.   T   F   Don't Know

30. Older persons who reduce their
    activity tend to be happier than those
    who do not.   T   F   Don't Know

31. When the last child leaves home, the
    majority of parents have serious
    problems adjusting to their
    "empty nest."   T   F   Don't Know

32. The proportion of widowed among
    the aged is decreasing.   T   F   Don't Know

Note. Adapted from *The Facts on Aging Quiz* (pp. 3–5 and 11–13) by E. B. Palmore with permission of Springer Publishing Company, Inc., © 1988.

THE IMPACT OF HOSPITALIZATION AND ILLNESS ON THE ELDERLY

The hospitalized elderly are at high risk for poor postdischarge outcomes. This means that they are more likely to experience unfortunate, and often preventable, events such as incontinence, reduced mobility, pressure ulcers, and delirium during and following their hospitalization. The frail elderly are also at increased risk of becoming more dependent on formal and informal care providers during and following their hospitalization.

One can use the "vicious cycle" model developed by Kuypers and Bengston (1986) to better understand how the hospital environment perpetuates dependence among the elderly population. Hospitalization can provoke a vicious cycle of dependency and permanent impairment among older people who have a multitude of chronic illnesses and who are minimally functional in a community or nursing home setting (Kuypers & Bengston, 1986). In some cases, diagnostic and treatment procedures meant to cure can trigger iatrogenic or nurisgenic conditions—negative reactions or results of medical or nursing treatment (Miller, 1975). The five steps of the vicious cycle of dependency follow.

Step One: Hospitalization for an Acute Episode of a Chronic Condition

Health problems, especially chronic illness, frequently limit the functional independence of older people, especially if an older person has two or more chronic conditions. As mentioned earlier, about 50% to 70% of those 65 or older have at least two or more chronic conditions (Guralnick, La Croix, & Everett, 1989). According to Schick (1986) the most common chronic conditions affecting those 65 years and older include—in descending order—arthritis, hypertension, heart disease, and hearing impairment.

Step Two: Treated as "Unable to" and Subsequent Dependence in the Hospital

Health professionals' may harbor biases toward older individuals. It is important to understand that there are certain myths, beliefs, and attitudes we hold that influence the way we treat the elderly. Most noninstitutionalized elderly are functionally competent; that is, they can perform all activities needed to care for themselves.

Second, family's fears and feelings about the patients' health and ability to care for themselves often lead families to assume duties and roles that patients would be more than willing and able to assume. More will be said on family fears and feelings in chapter 4.

Third, society has low expectations for elderly performance after hospital discharge and in general. This is, again, related to a common misconception about the elderly. Because they are old and frail, many do not expect them to perform well after hospitalization.

Fourth, hospitals may have unfamiliar and difficult routines. A hospital environment is designed for efficient delivery of acute care services, which may require the older person to relinquish some independent functions. In addition, the environment may be overwhelming to the elder (noise levels, lighting intensities, odors, cramped spacing, lack of privacy, visual images of highly technical equipment, lack of personalization, etc.) and can affect the elder's usual functional ability.

Step Three: Support of Hospital Staff Fosters Dependent Behavior, Which Can Result in Loss of Previous Skills and Atrophy of Abilities

Labels, when attached, stick. Matteson and McConnell (1988, p. 484) recount an old joke that illustrates the point that aging is not illness: An 81-year-old woman visits her doctor because she has pain in her left knee. After rather briefly examining her, the doctor pats the patient on the head and says, "Now Mildred, you're 81 years old—what else can you expect at your age?" To which the patient replies, "Doctor, my right knee is as old as my left knee, and it does not hurt."

Hospitals take many "fall" precautions. Often our concerns about the safety of the patient supersede the patient's autonomy. Physical and pharmacological restraints certainly foster dependence by reducing mobility. In the acute care setting it may be necessary for the elderly patient to take certain risks in rehabilitation, if this means improving mobility and increasing independence. Fall injury prevention may be more appropriately addressed in ways other than restraining, such as encouraging diagnosis and treatment of underlying medical conditions associated with accidents. For example, properly fitted eyeglasses and adequate podiatric care could reduce the risk of falls. Provider education about the importance of treating vision, hearing, and foot conditions may also be appropriate (Tideiksaar, 1989). In the community, acute care nurses can work with the Visiting Nurses Association (VNA) and other local service organizations to see that environmental hazards are removed from the home.

Hospital staff make many efforts to keep patients from hurting themselves. Common injuries to the noninstitutionalized elderly include burns (this would also include smoke inhalation from house fires) and pedestrian injuries. The risk of injury to patients at home presents a particularly difficult dilemma for nurses in the discharge process; do they discourage the patient from activities such as cooking or walking through busy traffic intersections, at times against the wishes of the patient, to ensure safety?

It is important to note that there are certain environmental changes that can be made in the home and elsewhere to reduce risk of injury without requiring daily behavioral change on the part of elderly people. These include carpet installation, smoke alarms, appropriate lighting, lower temperature settings on hot water heaters, etc.

Nurses give baths and medications. Nursing tasks, schedules, control, and service orientation further place the elderly patient in a dependent position. Studies have demonstrated that task-oriented nursing units promote dependent patient behavior, whereas individual-oriented nursing units promote independent patient behaviors (Miller, 1985). In the former, nurses become more preoccupied with tasks than rehabilitation of the individual patient.

Physicians make decisions about patients' health and future. Submission to authority further evodes the patient's sense of autonomy.

Step Four: Permanent Impairment and Incompetence

Elders may develop learned helplessness. Originally described by Seligman (1975), learned helplessness develops when individuals learn that their efforts will not produce results. Individuals perceive that they have little control over the events in their lives and eventually may become depressed.

One way to guard against learned helplessness is to allow patients to participate in the discharge planning process with the hospital staff and their family or supports. These team conferences let the patient set goals for himself or herself and ask questions of others on the team.

Elders may be discharged without a rehabilitation plan or program. Numerous studies have demonstrated that efforts at rehabilitation should be pursued because older people have the potential for recovery and should not be excluded from rehabilitation programs simply because of age. Older patients, even the very old and mentally compromised, benefit from rehabilitation in hospital settings (Schuman Beattie, Steed, Merry, Kraus, 1981; Applegate, Akins, Vanderzwaag, Thoni, & Baker, 1983; Parry, 1983; and Liem, Chernoff, & Carter, 1986). Major benefits were related to increased independent functioning and return to the pre-hospital setting.

Elders may be discharged as soon as possible. With the introduction of the Medicare prospective payment system based on diagnostic-related groups (DRGs), length of hospital stays for the elderly have been reduced. Therefore, patients are discharged "sicker and quicker" from the hospital (Knapp, 1986).

Step Five: Rehospitalization

Rehospitalization for another acute episode of chronic illness is likely to occur when patients are discharged more dependent than they were upon entering the hospital.

The elderly are susceptible to stereotypes. Stereotypes help us categorize incoming stimuli. They help us see how one group stands in relation to another. Health professionals, even gerontologists, may be guilty of stereotyping. *Ageism* influences the attitudes of health care professionals and policy makers in their treatment of the elderly. Ageism has been defined by Butler (1975, p. 12) as: "A process of systematic stereotyping of and discrimination against people because they are old. . . . Ageism allows the younger generations to see older people as different from themselves; thus they subtly cease to identify with their elders as human beings."

The outcome of the entire cycle may be dire: Reduced reserve and homeostatic capacity of older people predisposes them to increased morbidity during acute hospitalization or from trauma, major surgery, or administration of medication (Kohn & Monnier, 1987).

IMPROVING DISCHARGE PLANNING PROCEDURES

A recent study of the Prospective Payment System demonstrated that the number of patients discharged in unstable condition has increased across the board rather than in any specific patient or hospital subgroup (Rogers et al., 1990). In addition, there is evidence to show that some elderly patients may be discharged from hospitals with care needs too complex for their families to handle alone (Johnson & Fethke, 1985; Naylor, 1986; Wolock, Schlesinger, Dinerman, & Seaton, 1987).

The Goals of Discharge Planning

As a result of recent changes in the nature of hospital stays for the elderly, health care providers must re-examine the concept of discharge planning. The goals of discharge planning are to help patients and their families find solutions to their health care problems, ensuring that patients (a) receive the most appropriate level of care, (b) remain in the hospital for the shortest length of time, (c) receive the highest level quality care and are not hospitalized unnecessarily, and (d) have a planned post hospitalization program to meet continuing care needs with the least restrictive options.

Discharge planning has become more than a vehicle for moving the patient from one care environment to another. Today, discharge planning considers care provided during and following hospitalization, involves high-quality patient care and sound patient management practices, and coordinates individual units and disciplines to mobilize the resources necessary to assure a timely discharge from one level of care to another. The plan itself should reinforce the gains made in the acute care setting, be tailored as much as possible to the patients' needs and wishes, and help the patient deal with the limitations imposed at the time of discharge by the health care system and the stresses and losses experienced as a result of illness and diagnosis.

Continuing care entails the coordination of services to patients throughout three phases of illness: prehospitalization, hospitalization, and posthospitalization. The prehospital phase of the care continuum is concerned with health maintenance and health prevention. It involves efforts to maintain health through exercise, proper diet, and so on. It also entails patient education around issues such as self-care, alcohol and drug abuse, elder and child abuse, and health care consumerism. In the acute care setting, nurses should provide appropriate assessment and management of patient conditions in order to improve patient outcomes at discharge. Regardless of where the patient is discharged—home, home with assistance, or alternative care facility—there should be some protocol for patient follow-up.

A Multidisciplinary Process

Discharge planning as modeled in Figure 1.2 is a multidisciplinary process in that it involves the cooperation and coordination of several teams of people inside and outside the hospital. The primary team is the multidisciplinary, interactive group of health care providers charged with the following responsibilities:

- To *assess* the patient for continuing care needs
- To *develop* a plan of care that can enable the patient to move toward an optimal level of functioning
- To *implement* the plan of care

Because nurses are in a favorable position to assess the needs of the patient, they are valuable members of the multidisciplinary team. Physicians are important to the continuing care planning process because they communicate the ongoing, complex medical needs of the patient—a key component in planning the discharge. Social Service, a significant member of the multidisciplinary team, plays an important role in evaluating the emotional and environmental needs, the strengths, the limitations, the coping capacity, and the resource networks of the patient and the family. Other members of the primary team include the patients and the people close to them, and as necessary, physical, occupational, and speech therapists, and psychologists.

The resource team is a group of persons within the acute care setting who are available to the primary team as consultants for the patient's health care needs. These persons, trained in specialty health care fields, are used as resources and educators to the primary team. They assist in the implementation process as their expertise dictates.

The community team consists of persons from various community agencies and programs who are able to assist in the discharge planning process. The community team professionals continue in the community the plan of care that has been developed and carried out in the acute care setting. The essence of continuing care is established here when open communication is ongoing with the community team and when planning is an interdisciplinary team effort.

The nursing process provides a helpful framework for developing and implementing effective discharge plans (Zarle, 1987). *Assessment*

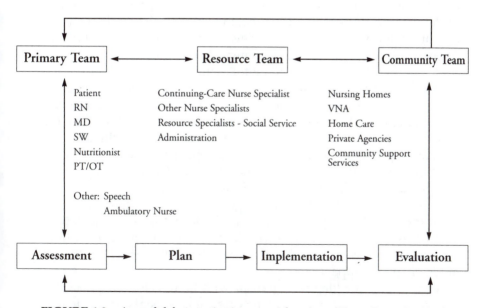

FIGURE 1.2   A model for continuing care planning. (*Note. From Continuing care: The process and practice of discharge planning* (p. 10) by N. C. Zarle, 1987, Rockville, MD: Aspen.)

involves collecting, validating, analyzing, and interpreting information about patients and their discharge environment. Beginning at admission, nurses should obtain information from patients, other professionals, and families.

At admission ask short-term patients (and all patients) the following questions (you may need to ask a patient spokesperson if they are unable to answer):

- Do you have health insurance?
- Where will you go when you leave the hospital?
- How will you get there?
- Do you have any family or friends who live with you or close to you?
- Who do you call on when you need transportation, food and shopping, cooking?

If the patient replies that he or she has no health insurance, no place to go after discharge, no way to get home, or no family and friends who can help with his or her care, ask what the patient's needs are related to housing, food and shopping, personal care, meal preparation, transportation, and housework. Then, begin to design the discharge plan. As you plan, communicate with relevant internal and external teams, project a discharge date, and document your actions.

For the longer term patient, the following factors may put the patient at risk for rehospitalization: age, living alone, no formal or informal support system, no financial support (i.e., no insurance nor financial reserves), current diagnosis, medical history (i.e., was the patient readmitted for the same diagnosis as in prior admissions?), nursing history (e.g., compliance with regime, pain management, coping skills, survival skills), environmental needs (e.g., housing, safety, equipment available), and projected discharge date.

Document your actions and findings in the patient record. Note that there are several strategies and tools available to assist documentation. (Examples of these tools from the Beth Israel Hospital in Boston, Massachusetts, are provided in Appendix B and C of this chapter and in the chapter 9 appendix.)

For the short- or long-term patient with high-tech needs, consider placement issues, complex home-care requriements, and dependence on community services. Also consider educational needs, long-term care placement options, and high-tech needs such as intravenous (IV) therapy (antibiotic/hydration), internal therapy, or respiratory ventilation).

Once this assessment is complete, ask yourself:

- Can the patient's discharge needs be met?
- Who will meet these needs? (Patient and/or family? With your help, or alone? With help from others, such as specialists, consultants, and community agencies?)

Planning involves the patient and the family in addressing their individual needs and desires for a continuing care plan. Using data gathered in the assessment, health care providers try to match patients with available resources based on patient eligibility and need. Planning requires flexibility and creativity, especially since the demands for continuing care services are rapidly increasing while resources seem to be decreasing.

Once you have identified the patient's needs, develop a plan. Ask yourself:

- What available resources do I have?
- Will the patient's insurance pay for this, and if so, how much?
- Has the patient used any community services prior to this admission?

Planning begins with your nursing diagnosis, which should guide your plan of action. Proceed through the following steps:

1. Provide hope, support, and freedom of choice to patients and their families.
2. Set goals with patients and families.
3. Evaluate yourself by asking: Is the plan timely? Is the plan appropriate for the patient's level? Is the plan realistic?
4. Document the care plan in the medical record, and communicate about it with everyone involved. If you only have time for a survival plan, take care of the most critical needs and move ahead with them.

Communicate appropriately and adequately. Remember that often in a time of stress people only hear what they want to hear. You can get very strange interpretations! So write the care plan down in the medical record and on paper for the patient.

Implementation involves arranging for services at home and acquiring the necessary equipment and supplies. It also may involve transferring the patient to another site such as a long-term care or rehabilitation facility. It is particularly important for providers in the acute care setting to communicate patient needs to those responsible for posthospital care.

Once the assessment and planning are complete and acceptable to all involved, implement the plan:

- Start patient and family education, keeping in mind that you may not be the one to complete it.
- Arrange for patient home care services, if necessary. Include equipment and supplies, follow-up appointments, and other services (e.g., adult day care, foster care, hospice transportation, appointments, sometimes housing, etc.).
- Arrange for transfer services (e.g., ambulance, cab, family pickup, train, airlines).
- Complete the patient referral form.
- Share information with relevant hospital staff, referral site staff, community resources, the patient, and his or her family.
- Give written discharge plan to the patient and to the family. They must sign it to show agreement and to acknowledge that they have received the plan and instructions.
- Record a brief summary discharge statement in the medical record.

Evaluation involves determining whether the patient's continuing care needs are being met. Evaluation often involves follow-up procedures to determine from patients, families, community agencies, and referral facilities whether the care and the services provided to the patient are satisfactory and delivered in a timely fashion. Evaluating the appropriateness of a continuing care plan can help to ensure the effectiveness of the future planning process for other patients who have similar needs.

There are three possible outcomes. Either (a) the patient remains at home, (b) the patient is moved to an alternative, facility or (c) the patient is readmitted within 30 days, within 14 days, or within 5 days. Follow this quick, but valuable and reliable preliminary evaluation with a telephone call 24 hours after the patient's first service-request provision. Evaluate the functional capacity of the individual, nursing and other care needs, and the ability of the service provider and family to meet the needs of the elderly individual after discharge.

Developing Action Plans to Improve Discharge Planning: Part I

Develop an action plan for improving discharge planning at your institutions. In Part I of the action plan, you will identify problems associated with discharge planning for the elderly at your institution and define an overall vision or goal related to that problem. The early phase of action planning involves identifying personal strengths and weaknesses that might affect one's abilities to implement a given plan, describing the most important issues or problems relating to discharge planning for the elderly, picking the single most important issue, and writing a vision statement related to this issue or problem. A copy of the action plan worksheet is included in Appendix D.

You will have the opportunity to complete and revise the different sections of your action plan throughout the book. Plans will vary depending on the needs and problems at a specific institution. The following sample case summaries, developed during the *Discharge Planning* field test, can suggest how to begin.

Example 1.   *Creating an Assessment Instrument to Improve Communication*

A floor nurse wants to provide information to all nurses regarding the importance of their primary role in discharge planning at her hospital. To attain her goal she has introduced a type of checklist or assessment instrument nurses could use to facilitate better communication regarding a specific patient in continuing-care rounds. She has planned to brainstorm with all members of the continuing-care team to see what information they have needed most or find most helpful. She expects to complete her project in one or two years with assistance from all members of the continuing care team.

Example 2. *Improving Interdisciplinary Communication Between Social Workers and RNs, Creating a Role for Nurses in Discharge Planning*

Another nurse's vision is increased involvement of primary nurses in discharge planning. In conjunction with the social worker, the primary nurse has participated in family meetings to review assessment findings and assist families in planning appropriate support systems.

This nurse sees implementation occurring in three phases: (a) ongoing discussion with the social work department about nursing's contribution to discharge planning, with an emphasis on nursing assessment of discharge needs; (b) education for nurses about aftercare options and placement services; and (c) nurse–family meetings during hospitalization at several points, including after admission, at discharge planning, and shortly before discharge.

This nurse estimates that it would take her one year to implement her action plan. For assistance she is consulting her nursing supervisor to facilitate meetings with social work. The nursing education department and the hospital discharge planning coordinator can arrange the appropriate access to discharge materials.

Example 3. *Designing and Implementing a Program to Improve Competency-Based Caring for the Elderly Patient*

A third nurse envisions improved gerontological nursing at her institution. Her strategy for realizing this vision is to design a competency-based caring program to become a part of the elder patient's orientation. Steps for instituting this program include: (a) auditing charts to identify when discharge planning was first addressed, (b) administering a survey for all RNs caring for elders, (c) developing a competency-based program on the care of the elder patient, (d) pilot-testing the program, (e) providing the program to all new RNs, and (f) re-evaluating the program.

This nurse estimates that the program will take her one to two years to develop and administer—three months for the audit, designing the survey and collecting the data, another three to six months to analyze the data and develop the program, three months to pilot and analyze, and another three months to make changes and implement the program.

For assistance in planning and implementing the program, she has consulted the nurse manager, the staff educator, geriatric nurse specialist, and other concerned RNs from the hospital.

Example 4. *Developing a Preadmission Screening Program*

A nurse manager wants to improve preadmission review so that she and her staff will be able to anticipate patients' needs better and manage cases more effectively. Her first strategy is to develop a preadmission screening program to ensure more comprehensive and appropriate hospital discharge planning. She has noted that patients who come into the preadmission lab have better post-discharge outcomes (e.g., are better matched with appropriate community services and are less likely to be readmitted shortly after discharge) than those who come in for the preoperative night. In fact, nursing staff have been able to predict, with preadmission data, when the patient will be back. Knowing what causes patient rehospitalization allows nurses to intervene prior to admission through appropriate discharge planning.

The nurse manager's second strategy for improving patient needs assessment and case management is to involve social workers in the assessment process. Her third strategy is to organize an in-service with staff nurses on their role in discharge planning. She has offered this in-service during the discharge planning rounds and has posted a suggestion box so that nurses could add their questions. As a fourth strategy, she plans to create a new flow sheet for functional assessment to assure consistent care provided by different nursing staff.

She plans to complete her action plan in one year and implement her changes unit by unit.

Example 5. *Improving Knowledge and Skill*

A fifth nurse has worked in continuing care for a long time. Yet, she has had no formal education in continuing care because there was no formal education system available in that area until recently. Her vision is issue oriented. She wants to improve communication and education related to discharge planning and continuing care by setting up a continuing care bulletin board on each floor. She plans to work with and monitor staff so that they would complete discharge plans on all patients (i.e., actually write a discharge plan). In addition, she wants to work closely with the hospital ethics committee—something her staff and department have never done before—when dealing with risky discharges. She estimates that these activities will take her between six months to a year to have in place.

SUMMARY

The key points of this chapter are:

1.   The introduction of the Prospective Payment System has drastically changed the nature of hospital stays for the elderly. They are being discharged "sicker and quicker."

2.   The concept of discharge planning has changed as a result of recent changes in health care reimbursement. Discharge planning has become more comprehensive, considering care provided during and following hospitalization and involving the coordination and cooperation of several teams of people both inside and outside the acute care setting.

3.   Nurses involved in discharge planning are in a position to guard and facilitate patients' rights to participate in decisions about their care and to help patients find the right balance between dependency and independence.

4.   The elderly are more likely to experience adverse, and often preventable, events during and following hospitalization.

5.   Even though the elderly may present multiple and chronic problems, most are capable of continuing normal activity.

CLINICAL EXERCISE

Describe the existing discharge planning model at your institution. Consider and describe (a) institutional formats for discharge planning, (b) individuals participating in the discharge planning process, (c) the person responsible for discharge planning, and (d) the role of the bedside nurse in the discharge planning process.

REFERENCES

Anderson, G. F., & Steinberg, E. P. (1984). Hospital re-admissions in the Medicare population. *New England Journal of Medicine, 311,* 1349–53.

Applegate, W. B., Akins, D., Vanderzwaag, R., Thoni, K., & Baker, M. G. (1983). A geriatric rehabilitation and assessment unit in a community hospital. *Journal of the American Geriatrics Society, 31,* 206–210.

Butler, R. (1975). *Why survive? Growing old in America.* New York: Harper & Row.

Callahan, D. (1987). *Setting limits: Medical goals in an aging society.* New York: Simon & Schuster.

Coulton, C. J., Dunkle, R. E., Hang, M., Chow, J., & Vielhaber, D. P. (1989). Locus of control and decision making for post-hospital care. *The Gerontologist, 29,* 627–632.

Eberle, C. M., & Besdine, R. W. (1992). Disease in old age. In T. T. Fulmer, & M. K. Walker (Eds.), *Critical care nursing of the elderly* (pp. 48–60). New York: Springer.

Fulmer, T., Ashley, J., & Reilly, C. (1986). Geriatric nursing in acute settings. *Annual Review of Gerontology and Geriatrics, 6,* 27–80.

Gottlieb, G. (1989). Optimizing mental functions of the elderly. In R. Lavizzo-Mouray, S. Day, D. Disereus, & J. A. Grisso (Eds.), *Practicing prevention for the elderly* (pp. 153–166). Philadelphia: Hanley & Belfus.

Guralnick, J. M., LaCroix, A. Z., & Everett, D. F. (1989). *Aging in the eighties: The prevalence of comorbidity and its association disability. Advance data from vital and health statistics* (No. 170). Hyattsville, MD: National Center for Health Statistics.

Johnson, H., & Fethke, C. (1985). Post-discharge outcomes and care planning for the hospitalized elderly. In E. McClelland, K. Kelly, & K. C. Bucknater (Eds.), *Continuity of care: Advancing the concept of discharge planning* (pp. 229–240). Orlando, FL: Grune & Stratton.

Knapp, M. T. (1986). Filling the gaps in health care: A hospital-based skilled nursing facility. *Nursing Management, 11,* 19–21.

Kohn, R. R., & Monnier, B. M. (1987). Normal aging and its parameters. In C. G. Swift (Ed.), *Clinical pharmacology in the elderly* (pp. 3–30). New York and Busel: Marcel Dekker.

Kuypers, J. A., & Bengston, U. L. (1986). Perspectives on the older family. In B. H. Giduz, T. L. Snow, C. J. Sanchez, et al. *Geriatric first aid kit* (p. vii). Chapel Hill, NC: Program on Aging, University of North Carolina School of Medicine.

Liem, P. H., Chernoff, R., and Carter, W. J. (1986). Geriatric rehabilitation unit: A three-year outcome evaluation. *The Journals of Gerontology, 41,* 44–50.

Matteson, M. A., & McConnell, E. S. (Eds.) (1988). *Gerontological nursing: Concepts and practice.* Philadelphia: Saunders.

Mezey, M. D., Rauckhorst, L. H., & Stokes, S. A. (1993). *Health assessment of the older individual.* New York: Springer Publishing Co.

Miller, A. A. (1975). Iatrogenic and nurisgenic effects of prolonged immobilization of the ill aged. *Journal of the American Geriatrics Society, 23,* 360–369.

Miller, A. A. (1985). A study of the dependency of elderly patients in wards using different methods of nursing care. *Age and Ageing, 14,* 132–138.

Naylor, M. (1986). *The health status and health care needs of older Americans* (Serial No. 99-L). Washington, DC: U.S. Senate Special Committee on Aging.

Palmore, E. (1988). *The facts on aging quiz.* New York: Springer Publishing Co.

Parry, F. (1983). Physical rehabilitation of the old, old patient. *Journal of the American Geriatrics Society, 31,* 482–484.

Prospective Payment Assessment Commission. (1989). *Medicare prospective payment and the American health care system.* Report to Congress. Washington, DC: Author.

Prospective Payment Assessment Commission. (1992). *Medicare prospective payment and the American health care system.* Report to Congress. Washington, DC: Prospective Payment Assessment Commission.

Rogers, W. H., Draper, D., Kahn, K. L., Keeler, E. B., Rubenstein, L. V., Kosecoff, J., & Brook, R. H. (1990). Quality of care before and after implementation of the DRG-based prospective payment system. A summary of effects. *Journal of the American Medical Association, 264,* 1989–1994.

Rowe, J. W., & Kahn, R. L. (1987). Human aging: Usual and successful. *Science, 237,* 143–149.

Schick, F. (Ed.) (1986). *Statistical handbook on aging Americans.* Phoenix, AZ: Oryz.

Schuman, J. E., Beattie, E. J., Steed, D. A., Merry, G. M., & Kraus, A. S. (1981). Geriatric patients with and without intellectual dysfunction: Effectiveness of a standard rehabilitation program. *Archives of Physical Medicine and Rehabilitation, 62,* 612–618.

Seligman, M. (1975). *Helplessness: On depression, development, and death.* San Francisco: Freeman.

Smith, D. M., Weinberger, M., Katz, B. P., & Moore, P. S. (1988). Postdischarge care and readmissions. *Medical Care, 26,* 699–708.

Staab, A. S., & Lyler, M. A. (1990). *Manual of geriatric nursing.* Glenview, IL: Scott Foresman.

Tideiksaar, R. (1989). *Falling in old age: Its prevention and treatment.* New York: Springer Publishing Co.

U.S. House of Representatives Subcommittee on Human Services of the Select Committee on Aging. (1987). *Exploding the myths: Caregiving in America.* Washington, DC: U.S. Government Printing Office.

U.S. Senate Special Committee on Aging. (1986). *Aging America: Trends and projections* (1985–86 ed.) Washington, DC: U.S. Government Printing Office.

Warshaw, G. A., Moore, J., Friedman, S. W., Currie, C. T., Kennie, D. C., Kane, W. J., & Mears, P. A. (1982). Functional disability in the hospitalized elderly. *Journal of the American Medical Association, 28,* 847–850.

Wolock, I., Schlesinger, E., Dinerman, M., & Seaton, R. (1987). The post-hospital needs and care of patients: Implications for discharge planning. *Social Work and Health Care, 12,* 61–76.

Zarle, N. C. (1987). *Continuing care: The process and practice of discharge planning.* Rockville, MD: Aspen.

SUGGESTED READINGS

Naylor, M. D. (1992). The implications of discharge planning for hospitalized elders. In T. T. Fulmer & M. K. Walker (Eds.), *Critical care nursing of the elderly* (pp. 331–347). New York: Springer Publishing Co.

APPENDIX A: Quiz Items and Answers

1. *People between the ages of 65 and 85 constitute the fastest growing age group in the United States.* <u>False</u>. According to the U.S. Bureau of the Census, people over 65 represented about 4% of the total U.S. population around the turn of the century. Today, people over 65 represent about 12% of the population, with the most rapid growth in the oldest group, over the age of 85 years. The percentage of individuals over the age of 65 years is expected to increase to 13% in the year 2000 and 22% by 2050. Two reasons for this growth are that people live longer and families have fewer children (Callahan, 1987).

2. *Health care costs for the elderly are increasing at the same rate that the elderly population itself is increasing.* <u>False</u>. Health care costs are rising much more dramatically than the number of elderly in the population.

According to a 1987 report presented to the Select Committee on Aging of the United States House of Representatives, the growth of the aged population has been accompanied by an astronomical increase in the health care costs for older persons. For example, in 1984, the 65-and-over age group represented 12% of the population but accounted for approximately 31% of total personal health care expenditures. And despite recent efforts to control costs, home health care expenditures for elderly patients increased 583% from 1980 to 1991 (Prospective Payment Assessment Commission, 1992).

3. *Almost half of all the money spent on health care for the elderly is for inpatient care in short-stay hospitals.* True. Warshaw and others (1982) found that older individuals use the services of short-stay hospitals more frequently and for longer periods than any other age group. They assert that the rate of hospitalization, the number of days of hospitalization per 1,000 persons, and the average length of stay all increase with age. Today, hospitalizations of Medicare beneficiaries account for at least one-quarter of all hospital admissions (Prospective Payment Assessment Commission, 1989; Anderson & Steinberg, 1984; Smith, Weinberger, Katz, & Moore, 1988).

4. *Among the elderly who require long-term care services, the vast majority live in the community rather than nursing homes or other long-term care facilities.* True. Only 20% of the elderly with long-term care needs live in nursing homes. The majority continue to live in the community primarily because of the unpaid assistance provided by family, friends, and neighbors. Even impaired elderly with serious health needs are cared for by members of their informal network. Approximately 75% of the noninstitutionalized impaired elderly rely solely on informal care. Only 5% receive all their care from paid sources (U.S. House of Representatives Subcommittee on Human Services of the Select Committee on Aging, 1987). It is important to also note that family care is one of the most critical factors in preventing or delaying nursing home utilization (U.S. House of Representatives Subcommittee on Human Services of the Select Committee on Aging, 1987).

5. *Most people become senile if they live long enough.* False. Most older people are not senile; that is, they do not have defective memory, nor are they disoriented or demented. A review of the literature by Palmore (1988) reveals that psychopathology among the aged is not common: Less than 10% of elderly individuals (age 65 and over) have significant or severe mental illness and another 10% to 32% have mild

to moderate mental impairment; but the majority are without impairment. Nevertheless, older people have good reason to be concerned about their mental health. More than 18% of older people are thought to experience significant mental health problems at any given time, and the incidence of altered mental functioning increases substantially in older age (Gottlieb, 1989).

6. *Alzheimer's disease (progressive senile dementia) is the most common type of chronic cognitive impairment among the aged.* True. The two most commonly diagnosed true dementias are Alzheimer's disease, which accounts for 50% to 70% of all dementias, and multi infarct dementia (Mezey, Rauckhorst, & Stokes, 1993). Mezey et al. (1993) also note that appropriate assessment and early identification of symptoms of mental and emotional disorders is important because it can lead to a more complete work-up, improved treatment, and referral to appropriate resources at discharge.

7. *Many of the disabilities of the elderly that used to be associated with the aging process are now understood to be the direct effects of illness.* True. Many changes previously attributed solely to aging are now recognized as changes attributable to disease, to lifestyle choices such as diet, smoking, and alcohol habits; or to environmental and occupational exposure (as summarized in Eberle & Besdine, 1992; Rowe & Kahn, 1987; Butler, 1975).

It is important to note that this particular question has implications for nurses and the care they provide to older individuals. When health care providers assume that symptoms and changes in older individuals are associated with aging rather than disease, they may fail to consider and apply therapeutic regimens that might reverse the symptoms and eventually lead to patient recovery.

8. *A person's height tends to decline in old age.* True.

9. *More older persons (65 or over) have chronic illnesses that limit their activity than do younger persons.* True. Four out of five community-dwelling elderly have at least one chronic condition; 50% to 70% have two or more chronic conditions (Guralnick, LaCroix, & Everett, 1989).

10. *Older persons have more acute (short-term) illnesses than do younger persons.* False.

11.   *Older persons have more injuries in the home than younger persons.*
<u>False</u>.

12.   *Older workers have less absenteeism than do younger workers.* <u>True</u>.

13.   *The life expectancy at age 65 of African Americans is about the same as Caucasians'.* <u>True</u>.

14.   *Men's life expectancy at age 65 is about the same as women's.*
<u>False</u>.

15.   *Medicare pays over half of the medical expenses for the aged.* <u>False</u>. According to the U.S. Senate Special Committee on Aging (1986), Medicare paid about 49% of the elderly's medical expenses in 1984.

16.   *Social Security benefits automatically increase with inflation.* <u>True</u>. Since 1975 Social Security benefits have automatically increased whenever the Consumer Price Index of the Bureau of Labor Statistics for the first quarter of a calendar year exceeds by at least 3% the index for the first quarter of the preceding year (Palmore, 1988).

17.   *Supplemental Security Income (SSI) guarantees a minimum income for needy aged.* <u>True</u>.

18.   *The aged do not get their proportionate share of the nation's income.*
<u>False</u>.

19.   *The aged have higher rates of criminal victimization than younger persons.* <u>False</u>.

20.   *The aged are more fearful of crime than are younger persons.* <u>True</u>.

21.   *The aged are the most law abiding of all adult age groups.* <u>True</u>.

22.   *There are about equal numbers of widows and widowers among the aged.* <u>False</u>: There are over five times more widows than widowers (Schick, 1986).

23.   *More of the aged vote than any other age group.* <u>False</u>.

24.   *There are proportionately more older persons in public office than in the total population.* <u>True</u>.

25.   *The proportion of African Americans among the aged is growing.*
<u>True</u>.

26.   *Participation in voluntary organizations (churches and clubs) tends to decline among the healthy aged.* <u>False</u>.

27.   *The majority of old people live alone.* <u>False</u>. Sixty-seven percent of the noninstitutionalized elderly live in family setings (Staab & Lyler, 1990).

28.   *The aged have a lower rate of poverty than the rest of the population.* <u>True</u>.

29.   *The rate of poverty among aged African Americans is about 3 times as high as among aged Caucasians.* <u>True</u>.

30.   *Older persons who reduce their activity tend to be happier than those who do not.* <u>False</u>.

31.   *When the last child leaves home, the majority of parents have serious problems adjusting to their "empty nest."* <u>False</u>.

32.   *The proportion of widowed among the aged is decreasing.* <u>True</u>. I appears that increasing longevity increases the average age at widowhood and thus increases the proportion of years beyond 65 in which both partners in a couple survive (Palmore, 1988).

APPENDIX B: Patient Admission Questionnaire

Name _____ Date _____ Room _____

1. Where will you go when you leave the hospital?

2. How will you get there?

3. Do you have family or close friends who live with you and assist with your transportation, shopping, cooking, etc.?

   Yes ____ No ____

4. If the answer to the above is no, indicate what is needed by circling the letters below:

   a. Housing   e. Transportation
   b. Food and shopping   f. Housework
   c. Personal care   g. Special Equipment
   d. Meal preparation   h. Other

5. Additional comments or concerns about going home:

_____

Primary Nurse

_____

Physician

Note. From *Continuing care: The process and practice of discharge planning* (p. 57) by N. C. Zarle, 1987, Rockville, MD: Aspen.

APPENDIX C: Initial Discharge Planning Sheet

Patient Admitted From:

M. D.	**RISK FACTORS** **DISCHARGE PLANS:** AGE - 70 YRS + YES NO PROJECTED LEVEL OF CARE LIVES ALONE YES NO LEVEL PRIOR TO ADMISSION _____ HEALTH INSURANCE YES NO EXPECTED DISCHARGE STATUS SUPPORT SYSTEM YES NO _____ **PROJECTED DISCHARGE DATE:** INSTRUCTIONS/CONCERNS: (i.e., Rehabilitation, skilled Nursing Needs, etc.) Initials

RISK FACTORS

AGE - 70 YRS +   YES   NO

LIVES ALONE   YES   NO

HEALTH INSURANCE   YES   NO

SUPPORT SYSTEM   YES   NO

DISCHARGE PLANS:

PROJECTED LEVEL OF CARE

LEVEL PRIOR TO ADMISSION _____

EXPECTED DISCHARGE STATUS

_____

PROJECTED DISCHARGE DATE:

INSTRUCTIONS/CONCERNS: (i.e., Rehabilitation, skilled Nursing Needs, etc.)

Initials

PRIMARY NURSE

ANY ANTICIPATED PROBLEMS AT DISCHARGE (if yes, state why)

Initials

SOCIAL WORK

CONSULT REQUESTED BY _____   DATE _____

SPECIAL PROBLEMS   _____

Patient Screened By	Accepted	Rejected	Anticipated Date of Discharge
1. _____	_____	_____	_____
2. _____	_____	_____	_____
3. _____	_____	_____	_____

OTHER COMMENTS

Source: Beth Israel Hospital, Boston, MA

APPENDIX D: Action Plan Worksheet*
Part I—Vision Statement

Name: _____

Work Address: _____
_____
_____

Three major strengths I bring to my job are:

1. _____
2. _____
3. _____

Three major areas where I want to improve my skills related to discharge planning are:

1. _____
2. _____
3. _____

The four most important issues or problems related to discharge planning for the elderly at my institution that I feel I need to address now are:

1. _____
2. _____
3. _____
4. _____

The single most important issue or problem related to discharge planning for the elderly at my institution that I feel I need to address now is:

_____
_____
_____
_____

* *Note*: The Action Plan Worksheet was adapted from one originally developed by Christine Blaber, MEd, and Kimberly Dash, MPA, Education Development Center, Inc., under a grant from the U.S. Department of Education.

Describe the situation:

_____

_____

_____

_____

My vision statement related to this issue or problem is:

_____

_____

_____

_____

_____

Chapter 2

DEVELOPING COMMUNICATION SKILLS FOR BETTER DISCHARGE PLANNING

LEARNING OBJECTIVES

At the end of this chapter readers will be able to:

1. Practice and improve your communication skills with elderly patients based on an understanding of communication theory and sound gerontological practices
2. Perform a practice exercise in communication skills with an elderly patient
3. Identify several ways to improve communication with health care professional within your home institution and in the community

This chapter covers ways in which good communication, whether between patient and provider or among members of the multidisciplinary discharge team, is essential to the continuing care process.

The chapter begins with a critique of a sample nurse–patient dialogue, pointing out effective and ineffective communication methods. A discussion follows on general strategies for communicating with the elderly and, in particular, elderly from diverse backgrounds.

The second half of the chapter focuses on the importance of multidisciplinary communication in the continuing care process. The various teams and resources involved in the communication process and methods and forums of communication are described. A second case illustrates ways nurses can resolve patient issues using multidisciplinary communication methods.

COMMUNICATING WITH ELDERLY PATIENTS

Establishing rapport with patients is one of the key elements in the communication process. By doing so, the nurse is better able to elicit the type of information that is relevant to the discharge planning process.

Refer to the case, your first visit with Mr. Jones, and think about what was done "right" and what was done "wrong" in the case. How could the nurse's approach to communication or data gathering have been more effective? In what ways, if any, was it effective? Think about ways you initiate and maintain communication with your elderly patients and how your experience is relevant to this case.

Your First Visit with Mr. Jones

You are a nurse working on unit 3 and have a new patient in room 302. Mr. Jones is an 82-year-old patient admitted during the previous day with "fever of unknown origin." The report you receive states that he has been demanding and complaining since admission.

You enter his room, introduce yourself and explain that you will be caring for him today. Then you ask him, "How are you feeling today, Mr. Jones?"

Mr. Jones sighs, wrings his hands, raises his eyebrows and responds that he thinks he is feeling fine today.

You notice that Mr. Jones's facial expression and actions do not match his message and you say, "You seem a little anxious."

After some silence, Mr. Jones tells you that he is distressed and suddenly blurts out: "All my daughter-in-law cares about is money!"

This sounds like a touchy subject and you are uncertain about whether or not to pursue it. So you ask, "Do you not get along with your daughter-in-law?"

Mr. Jones is silent for a while, then just shrugs his shoulders. For now this subject seems off limits to you, so you decide to take another approach. You ask about his home, since you noticed in his admission records that he lives alone: "So, I hear you live on Walnut Street. How do you like living there?"

Mr. Jones seems to appreciate the change in topic and talks at some length about how he really likes his house and his neighborhood. You learn that he has lived there for 40 years or so. You also find that he is a man who appreciates his independence. He says that he has grown accustomed to doing things his own way and would find it hard to adapt to another person's rules.

You then ask him whether or not he has any concerns about living alone. He says that he has none and receives regular visits from a visiting nurse, which take care of all his health worries.

You ask him what he would do if he became too weak or sick to take care of himself, or even worse, if he were to fall terribly ill between nursing visits. This question seems to annoy Mr. Jones. He is silent for some time, and then finally answers that he is tired and does "not want to talk about this stuff anymore." You decide to adhere to his wishes and let yourself out the door.

Questions to Consider

1. How do you feel about the things that the patient said? What do you think the patient is concerned about? How do your own beliefs about older people, aging, family relationships, and money affect the communication process? What are the hardest issues for you to face (e.g., "all my daughter-in-law thinks about is money")?

2. How do you define yourself within this situation? How do you view your role as helper? Advocate? Supporter? Communicator? Clinician? What are the responsibilities and limits of your role?

3. What type of information is appropriate to discharge planning and what is not? How much information should you collect?

4. How does the environment affect the communication exchange?

5. How do the needs and concerns of the hospitalized elder affect the communication process? What are some of the special needs and

concerns of the hospitalized elder that you have witnessed in your practice? Keep in mind, for example, the physiological changes of normal aging, such as difficulty discriminating sounds when there is more than one sound and reductions in visual acuity.

6. What are some ways to initiate conversation with elderly patients in order to establish rapport?

7. How do you elicit information from elderly patients that will be helpful to you in planning for discharge and continuing care? What kinds of questions are conversation stoppers instead of openers? What ways have you tried to communicate verbally and nonverbally with the elderly? What works? What does not?

An Introduction to Patient–Provider Communication

The goal of effective communication is to ensure that sufficient knowledge of patient needs is obtained to effectively plan care and develop discharge plans. The better informed a nurse is about a patient, the more individualized the discharge plan. The process of gathering information should start at admission and continue throughout the hospitalization period.

Communication can be defined as:

- A complex, dynamic interchange of verbal and nonverbal messages and meanings between people
- The means whereby information is transferred
- The process of imparting knowledge
- A social process
- Something continuous and fluid

During any given communication, the roles of participants, messages relayed, and meanings implied develop, change, and grow.

A communication model has at least four components. Each part is influenced by a variety of factors that in turn influence the quality of the communication process. The first component is the *sender*, either nurse or patient, who transmits the communication message. Many factors influence the sender: personal background, attitudes, values, beliefs, and knowledge. The patient, for example, may feel that it is inappropriate to discuss personal and family problems with the nurse or physician. The nurse may have to try harder to make the patient feel more comfortable before discussing some of those personal problems. One solution is to talk about less sensitive issues first. For example, the nurse in the case misadvisedly asked Mr. Jones about a particularly sensitive issue, his relationship with his daughter-in-law, even though she knew the subject caused Mr. Jones discomfort.

The second element, the *message*, can be verbal or nonverbal. Try to observe facial expressions and notice arm and hand gestures. Often the verbal and nonverbal messages will be contradictory. For example, Mr. Jones claimed that everything was fine, yet was wringing his hands and sighing.

The third component, the *receiver*, is influenced by the same types of factors as the sender. As a receiver, the professional should actively listen to the sender, openly observe behavior and thus increase the likelihood that the message intending to be sent is the one that is being received.

The fourth component the *context* of the communication, is the environment in which the communication is occurring. The environment is defined by such factors as the illness of the patient, the cultural backgrounds of the communicants, their value systems, and their beliefs. Physical surroundings may also influence the communication process: Another person in the room may inhibit the patient; peripheral noises may distract him or her; and bright lighting may make the interview seem like an interrogation.

Factors Affecting Communication with the Elderly

Certain adaptive tasks may affect the communication process. Clark and Anderson (1967), define adaptive as learning to live in a particular way according to a particular set of values as one or as one's culture changes. They identify five adaptive tasks associated with aging:

- Recognition of aging and definition of instrumental limitations
- Redefinition of physical and social environment
- Substitution of alternate sources of need satisfaction
- Reassessment of criteria for evaluation of self
- Reintegration of values and life goals

The person who has successfully adapted to aging is able to adjust to the decremental changes while continuing to grow and contribute to his or her community. Those who do not adjust have difficulty in accepting their life style and difficulty in finding substitutes for the things that satisfy their needs. Attitudes and beliefs about aging may vary and nurses should be aware of how these affect their work with patients. For example, some believe that aging is a purely deteriorative process while others see it as a developmental process with both positive and negative aspects.

Physical changes and tolerances affect the communication process. The process of aging occurs at all levels: cellular, organic, and systemic. Loss of cells and loss of physiological reserve make up the dominant process of aging and are certainly issues in discharge planning. (Specific age-related factors will be reviewed in chapter 3.) While the degree of loss may vary from patient to patient, the nurse should take into account the patients' stamina and ability to endure lengthy interviews. If, for example, the patient is not alert or able to communicate his or her thoughts and feelings, information for discharge planning may be gathered from other sources, such as the family, medical records, other institutions such as nursing homes, Visiting Nurses Associations (VNAs), and home health care agencies.

The main effects of aging on communication are those that involve hearing and vision loss. The older person requires good lighting with less glare and certain tone alterations. Speech may be slower, but specific speech aphasias are the result of illness, not a normal outcome of aging. With aging, loss in acuity begins to affect hearing of sound in the higher frequency ranges (1,500 to 4,000 Hz) and gradually affects the lower frequencies (500 to 1,500 Hz). Background noise tends to exaggerate problems associated with hearing loss of high frequency sounds, especially for individuals with presbycusis (i.e., loss of ability to perceive or discriminate sounds as part of the aging process) (Corso, 1971).

The elderly require more time to absorb and integrate new information. This is particularly significant when nurses assume the role of educator. For example, nurses may find that in order to enhance patient compliance with medication, they need to make the messages short and simple, and repeat them.

The environment or social situation may need to be altered to enhance the communication process. In hospitalization, patients experience disruption of inclusion, control, and affection needs. Inclusion needs are fulfilled by associating and interacting with others. Through inclusion individuals gain feelings of significance and self-worth; they are distinguished from others, understood, and have others interested enough to seek and discover their particular likes and dislikes. Hospitalization for the elderly frequently undermines inclusion because it means displacement from family, friends, and loved ones who may not be able to visit them at the hospital.

The need for control is manifested by the ability to make decisions and assume responsibility for oneself. The hospital structure eliminates decision making from even the most menial tasks of daily living such as when to eat, when to get up, or go the bathroom. Nurses can assist patients in maintaining control by encouraging them to assume decision making for some parts of their own care.

Affection needs are usually met by the family, friends, and spouse. Without them the older person may turn to the nurse to confide anxieties, wishes, and feelings.

Occasionally, a change in the environment triggers a temporary confusional state that can impede nurse–patient communication. A patient recently moved to the hospital after suffering a fall or a heart attack may not know where he or she is and may not be too coherent. The nurse should approach any state of confusion in elderly persons as a temporary problem, and try to orient them to their environment.

General Communication Techniques

Nurses can help assure that elderly patients' needs and wishes are understood, if they are able to communicate effectively with them. Many factors can distort the message within a communication process, but specific techniques can be learned to lessen the frequency of misinterpretation. The nurse's role in communicating with patients is to gather information, to educate, and to offer support and reassurance. Some general techniques are described below.

Avoid using questions that will give you a "yes" or "no" answer. Nurses should work towards building a rapport with their patients in order to elicit background information that might be useful in the discharge planning process. When given the opportunity, most people like to talk about themselves and the things that are troubling them. Openended questions require time and convey the message that you care about the person and are sincerely interested. In addition, they tend to yield much more informative and rich responses from the patient than do closed-ended questions.

Ways in which open-ended questions can be prefaced include:

- What do you think about . . .
- Tell me about . . .
- How did you feel when . . .
- Describe what happened . . .
- Tell me what is your greatest concern right now . . .

However, avoid asking too many questions of this type because it can confuse and tire the patient by extending the interview.

Avoid using leading questions. Leading questions are the kinds of question that imply an expected answer, such as: "You would like to lose weight, wouldn't you?" or "Wouldn't you rather live with your son or daughter?" Rather, ask: "What would you like to weigh?" or "Where would you like to live?"

When appropriate, allow for periods of silence to prompt the patient to speak. If you find that you are doing most of the talking in the conversation, allow for moments of silence. Most people are uncomfortable with silence, so the patient will likely begin to talk with you. Silence gives older persons time to collect and organize their thoughts. Silence gives you time for closer observation of the elder. However, silence should convey an acceptance, not a stand-off. It may be possible that the person could not hear you, may not want to hear you, is no longer interested in the topic, is tired, or is thinking of the next thing to say. Also note that older people can take a longer time to process information.

Clarify ambiguous or confusing statements made by the elderly patient. For example, when "Ms. Josephs" tells you that she has no family to care for her, yet later begins talking about her son who lives 10 miles from her in the same town, you need to clarify this discrepancy. For example, her statement may mean that the son is unable or unwilling to help, or that Ms. Josephs does not feel comfortable making her needs known. You need to be sure you understand what the patient meant for you to understand.

Clarification can be accomplished in a variety of ways:

- Ask a question, such as: "What do you mean?" People will usually attempt to rephrase their statements so that you understand.
- Point out inconsistencies or omissions: "You told me about . . . , but you didn't say anything about . . ."

- Restate, in your own words, what you interpreted the patient to have said and ask if your interpretation is correct.
- Sometimes echoing back (i.e., using the patient's exact words) will encourage the patient to elaborate even further on a topic.
- Summarize what the conversation has been about and ask the patient if your summary is correct.
- Identify similarities and differences (e.g., "Yesterday you said you felt . . . , but today you are saying . . .").
- Ask the patient for an example of what he or she is saying.

When necessary, redirect the patient back to the topic at hand. Occasionally the patient will diverge from the topic. Let's say, for example, you would like "Mr. Rose" to elaborate on his relationship with his son, seeing its importance for planning continuing care after discharge. You want to find out whether or not the son will be a viable resource for his father's care. However, when asked about the relationship, Mr. Rose says only a few words and then begins to talk about raising his son, and from there gets sidetracked and begins talking about fishing trips they took together. You want to get back to the present relationship between father and son. One suggestion for redirecting the conversation: "That's very interesting and I want to hear more about it, but first finish telling me about your present relationship with your son."

Pay attention to nonverbal cues. They provide insight into how the patient is really feeling. Notice the patient's posture, facial expressions, and attention pattern. In Part A of the case study, for example, Mr. Jones's nonverbal gestures signaled that something was bothering him even though he said he was feeling fine.

Offer support and reassurance throughout the conversation. Throughout the exchange, answer questions, offer reassurances, and provide comfort. Communication is a two-way process and your active participation encourages the patient to open up more and provide the information needed to plan for continuing care. Also, provide an opportunity for the patient to ask questions: "I've asked you a lot of questions, are there any questions you would like to ask me?" When ending an exchange, summarize any problems that came out of the talk and any agreed-upon methods for dealing with the problem.

Recognize feelings and invite elder individuals to expand upon their feelings. Upon hearing negative feelings people often respond in a way that denies another's feelings. How often have you asked a co-worker, "How are you feeling today?" and replied to the response, "Just terrible," with, "Well, maybe you'll feel better tomorrow," or "Oh, I'm sorry to hear that," and then moved rapidly on your way? Such responses block further discussion. A better technique is to remain with the person and follow up with an open-ended question for clarification.

People also tend to change the subject when they feel uncomfortable with a topic. The statement by Mr. Jones, in Part A of the case study, that his daughter-in-law is only interested in money could cause many of us to change the topic. However, exploratory questions such as "What do you mean?" can encourage patients to talk more about what is bothering them. While some elderly patients may be more comfortable than others about expressing feelings, talking can help to dissipate frustration and may even lead to solutions. For example, once Mr. Jones's problem is defined, the nurse can help validate many of his feelings by pointing out that anger or frustration is normal under certain circumstances. The nurse also has obtained information relevant to Mr. Jones's discharge plan and continuing care.

There is often some anxiety among the hospitalized elderly on the issue of death and dying. Acknowledging feelings is especially important when exploring this issue. As the elderly try to adjust to the death of a spouse or even other elderly friends, they begin to realize their own mortality but may need help talking about their feelings about their own death.

Look for resources and successes in past experiences. Elderly people have years of rich experience and may share their memories for a variety of reasons. You can use this sharing of memories to enlarge your relationship with elders, to help them explore the memory in more detail, or to ask a question as a bridge to other information. Looking to the past may help the elder find a solution to a present-day dilemma.

Avoid treating the elderly patient as a child. The nurse, in a caregiver role, may inadvertently treat the older person as a child. Nurses may find that they often direct the older person in self-care needs, rather than allowing the old person to maintain decision making and autonomy. Family members, particularly adult children who experience some reversal of traditional parent–child roles, may also limit the older persons autonomy.

Convey respect. Demonstrating respect may be especially challenging when working with confused elders. Approach the confused patient with the assumption that they do want to function in reality and in the present. Orient the person to the present, explain procedures, and be specific and clear about what is expected. With other elders balance independence with dependence. Assess the patients' abilities and create an atmosphere wherein that elder can maintain as much independent function as possible. For example, focus on the person before beginning a task and ask before invading personal space. Also knock before entering a patient's room.

Rules for Communicating with Members of Diverse Groups

Today health care providers face the challenge of providing appropriate care to increasingly diverse consumer populations. In order to meet the needs of diverse groups in developing discharge plans, nurses must build their skills in cross-cultural communication. Kavanagh (1991, p. 198) describes essential goals for facilitating communication with members of diverse groups. We have adapted some of these goals and describe them below. You may note that many of these methods are similar to the general communication techniques listed above.

- Promote a feeling of acceptance.
- To the extent possible, establish open communication.
- Present yourself with confidence, shake hands if it is appropriate.
- Strive to gain the patient's trust, but do not resent it if you do not get it.
- Understand what members of the cultural or subcultural group consider as "caring," both attitudinally and behaviorally.
- Understand the relationship between the patient and authority figures.
- Understand the patient's desire to please and his or her motivation to comply or not comply.
- Anticipate diversity, and avoid stereotypes by sex, age, ethnicity, socioeconomic status, and other social categories.
- Avoid assumptions about where patients come from; let them tell you their origins instead. (Most people are pleased when others show sincere interest in them.)
- Understand the patient's goals and expectations.

- Make your goals realistic.
- Emphasize positive points and strengths of patients' health beliefs and practices.
- Distinguish and show proper respect for male and female decision makers.
- Know the traditional, health-related practices common to the group with whom you are working, and do not discredit any of the practices unless you know specific ones that are harmful.
- Try to make the setting comfortable; consider colors, music, atmosphere, scheduling expectations, seating arrangements, pace, tone, and other environmental variables.
- Whenever possible and appropriate, involve significant community leaders. Confidentiality is important, but the leaders know the issues affecting communication and often can suggest acceptable interventions.
- Respect values, beliefs, rights, and practices although some may conflict with your determination to make changes. Every group and individual wants respect above all else.
- Learn to appreciate the richness of diversity as an asset rather than as a hindrance to communication and effective discharge planning.

COMMUNICATING WITH THE MULTIDISCIPLINARY TEAM

Nurses must understand and be able to use the services provided within their institutional setting to establish an effective discharge plan for a patient. Understanding how the various community services operate will greatly enhance their ability to develop a realistic discharge plan.

The various teams and resources involved in discharge planning all participate in the communication process of continuing care. The primary team, the resource team, and the community team all work together not only in assessing the patient, but also in planning, implementing, and evaluating the discharge plan. Multidisciplinary communication is also a cyclical process—evaluation provides information that will be helpful in improving future discharge plans. The information below discusses how teams can enhance communication and thus improve patient outcomes at discharge.

Methods of Communication

Table 2.1 summarizes the procedures hospitals use to ensure communication. Internal communication involves communication among hospital staff and departments, and typically includes (a) referrals, (b) rounds and team conferences, and (c) nurses' documentation.

Referrals are probably the most common method of internal communication. In the case of a family dispute or suspicion that an elder is being physically abused, the nurse may want to consult the hospital social worker or the social service resource specialist. Or, if it is recommended that a patient will need some physical therapy before being discharged to the care of the family, then the physical therapist is asked to work on the case.

Conferences of the discharge planning team most likely include members of the primary team, for example, the patient, the family, the nurse, the physician, and in other cases members of the resource team, when appropriate.

Nursing documentation of patient assessment and current status is accomplished by means of assessment forms and screening tools. By carefully documenting the patient's functional, physical, and mental status, for example, the nurse helps ensure that others on the discharge planning team are likely to get the assessment information and apply it to the planning process.

External communication involves communication between hospital staff and outside agencies and organizations. Two types of external communication are (a) community referral forms and (b) community educational series.

Community referral forms are used to transfer specific information to community agencies. If, for example, a nurse believes that a particular patient is being abused, the nurse may need to send a referral form for that patient to social services.

Community educational services provided by hospitals or other agencies are outreach programs to help the community deal with the health care needs of the elderly and find ways to meet them. Some of these educational programs may deal with establishing independent living, preventing injuries, or learning about medications.

TABLE 2.1 Communication Forums

Internal Communication	
Type	*Purpose*
1. Continuing-care rounds	A multidisciplinary team meeting to identify patient care needs, set goals and objectives, and match services with needs
2. Family meetings	To create and implement a discharge plan that meets as many of the specific needs and requests of both patient and family as possible
3. Nursing rounds	To address care issues and continuing care needs
4. Other meetings	To involve other disciplines in planning continuing care of patients with multiple problems and/or, who are difficult to discharge
5. Various nursing communication	To document and relate patient assessment data
6. Discharge-related forms and summaries	To document patient continuing care needs
7. Patient chart documentation	To relate patient states and observations, actions taken in response to identified needs, and outcomes of actions
8. Nursing diagnosis	To identify those patients requiring continuing care
9. Educational series	To gather information on community resources available to the patient

External Communication	
Type	*Purpose*
1. Community referral forms	To transfer specific information to community agencies
2. Community educational series	To focus on the health care needs of the elderly and ways to meet them

Refer to the case, "A Later Visit with Mr. Jones." Keep in mind that once nurses are able to build rapport with patients and collect the information they need, they must then share that information with others. The case study is a continuation of the Mr. Jones story begun earlier in this chapter.

A Later Visit with Mr. Jones

You've now established some rapport with Mr. Jones. In your second meeting with him, he tells you that his daughter-in-law and his son want him to sell his house and move in with them. This upsets him and he places most of the blame for this request on his daughter-in-law: "All she wants is my money! She even wants me to pay rent!" he said.

His situation is further aggravated by his hospitalization and his prognosis. He thinks that his children will see this as an opportunity to take advantage of him. He says, "They'll never stop hounding me now that they see I'm sick! This is just the excuse they've been waiting for!" Mr. Jones has always prided himself on being able to take care of everything, even at his age, and does not think he will like living in his son's home. Mr. Jones's son has children of his own and Mr. Jones does not want to be a burden.

You later decide to approach Mr. Jones's son and daughter-in-law to find out, from their perspective, what they think about their father's continuing care. They tell you that they are quite concerned about his ability to take care of himself. They say that Mr. Jones often telephones them to make many requests: Could they pick up something for him from the market, could they fix the loose plank on the stairs, and so on. Mr. Jones's son says that he does not mind doing these things, but he is a busy man and lives about 15 miles away from his father. He thinks it might be easier on everyone if his father were to move in with him and his wife. The daughter-in-law said that they have never asked their father to sell his house. However, they feel that his capacity to take care of himself is diminishing quickly. With the onset of this recent illness, they feel quite certain that he should move in with them. When you ask them whether or not they would charge their father rent, they reply that this was something they had not decided, but that the answer would probably be no.

A few days later you find out by chance from the attending physician that Mr. Jones told him that it might not be a bad idea if he moved in with his son and daughter-in-law. In light of his recent illness, he was beginning to worry about living alone, keeping up his small home, and taking care of himself.

Questions to Consider

1. How would you use the information you've collected?

   Would you pass it on in a formal setting like staff rounds, or more informally?

2. Do you document your findings in the medical record?

3. What should you do with the information obtained from communicating with the patient? with the family? with the physician?

   How would you share this information?

4. How can the family help or hinder communication with the patient?

5. What problems might you experience working with other staff on discharge planning for patients?

6. How would you resolve turf issues among staff members?

7. How would you begin to mobilize support for a multi-disciplinary discharge planning process?

Although the nurse's role in discharge planning will vary from institution to institution, as will the models of discharge planning, interdisciplinary communication issues remain the same. Lack of communication forums, lack of documentation, and turf issues often impede the flow of information. Whether addressing the discharge needs of a specific patient or promoting an agenda of change (i.e., improving the discharge planning process), nurses need to identify institutional barriers to communication and ways they can overcome them. In the final chapters of this book, nurses will learn more about the processes of institutional assessment and change.

SUMMARY

The key points of this chapter are:

1. Effective nurse-patient communication requires knowledge of age-related needs and concerns.
2. Many factors can distort the communication process, but specific techniques can be applied to lessen the frequency of misinterpretation.
3. Various players, including individuals inside and outside the hospital, are involved in the communication process of continuing care.

CLINICAL EXERCISE

Use the Communication Assessment Sheet (see Appendix A at the end of Chapter 2) to describe ways in which you have applied some of the communication techniques learned in this chapter.

REFERENCES

Clark, M., & Anderson, P. B. (1967). *Culture and aging*. Springfield, IL: Charles C Thomas.

Corso, J. F. (1971). Sensory process and age effects in normal adults. *Journal of Gerontology, 26,* 90–105.

Kavanagh, K. H. (1991). Social and cultural influences: Values and beliefs. In J. L. Creasia, & B. Parker (Eds.), *Conceptual foundations of professional nursing practice* (pp. 167–210). St. Louis, MO: Mosby.

SUGGESTED READINGS

Bender-Dreher, B. (1987). *Communication skills for working with elders.* New York: Springer Publishing Co.

Cox, B. J., & Waller, L. (1987). *Communicating with the elderly.* St. Louis, MO: Catholic Health Association of the United States.

Kavanagh, K. H., & Kennedy, P. H. (1992). *Promoting cultural diversity: Strategies for health care professionals.* Newbury Park, CA: Sage.

APPENDIX A: Communication Assessment Sheet

Patient Name: **Date:**

1. Describe each of the following aspects of the environment.

    Location:

    Privacy:

    Interruptions:

    Background noise:

    Lighting:

    Temperature:

2. What was the state of the patient during the interchange?

    Comfort level and physiological needs:

    Ability to attend:

    Affect:

    Cognition:

3. What communication method(s) did you use? How did they work?

    Open-ended questions:

    Leading questions:

    Silence clarification:

    Redirection:

    Validation:

    Nonverbal gestures of attending:

    Touch:

    Other:

4. In general, how did the interchange go?

Chapter **3**

PATIENT ASSESSMENT

LEARNING OBJECTIVES

At the end of this chapter, readers will be able to:

1. Recognize the major physical, psychological, cognitive, and functional changes that occur during the normal aging process
2. Distinguish between the normal changes of aging and disease processes in elderly adults
3. Assess physical, mental, and functional status of elderly patients and make recommendations for continuing care based on these assessments
4. Improve collection of patient prehospital data
5. Develop a nursing protocol for the early identification and treatment of elderly at risk for poor postdischarge outcome
6. Teach patients new skills for adapting to functional disability and help them work towards new definitions of independence and support
7. Begin to match patients' needs with available resources

A patient assessment of discharge needs involves gathering information about (a) sociodemographics, (b) general health status, (c) functional status, (d) mental status, (e) self-esteem, (f) stress level, (g) perception of health status, (h) prehospitalization resource use, and (i) perceived resource needs after discharge (Naylor et al., 1994). Often nurses are responsible for collecting much of the information used to determine patient discharge needs. Therefore, it is crucial that they be aware of the factors affecting geriatric patient assessment and the advantages and disadvantages of certain methods of assessment.

Although other elements of the comprehensive geriatric assessment are mentioned, this chapter is devoted primarily to the physical, mental/emotional, and functional changes that occur with aging and how these affect assessment of older patients. (Chapters 4 and 5 provide greater detail on home, caregiver, and community assessment.) The chapter opens with a discussion of the factors that put the elderly at risk for poor postdischarge outcomes and how nurses can identify these factors through a comprehensive geriatric assessment.

The second part of this chapter is a discussion of the effects of normal aging on the physiological and functional processes of the elderly. It provides guidelines for the physical assessment with a brief review of systems, and of how physiological change associated with normal aging affects these systems.

Third, we focus on mental and emotional assessment. It provides information on the psychological changes that occur with aging, ways to assess these changes, and how these changes in status are relevant to discharge planning. Finally the importance of functional assessment and the utility of specific measures are described.

IDENTIFYING PATIENTS AT RISK FOR POOR POSTDISCHARGE OUTCOMES

The prevention of avoidable poor discharge outcomes should be a major focus of discharge planning for the hospitalized elderly (Naylor, 1992).

Some examples of poor postdischarge outcomes might include (a) repeat hospitalizations, (b) institutionalization, (c) declines in physical or mental health, (d) development of iatrogenic or nursigenic conditions, (e) increased reliance on community services, and (f) greater caregiver stress.

How can hospitals, and specifically nurses, improve geriatric postdischarge outcomes? In general, accurate patient assessment combined with prevention, management, and treatment of certain conditions can lead to improved patient outcomes.

One of the best ways to determine patient postdischarge needs and avoid poor patient outcomes is to conduct a thorough patient assessment. Table 3.1 reviews some of the components of patient assessment

TABLE 3.1   A Guide to Patient Assessment

Physical health

The patient's perception of the current illness and how he or she believes it will affect lifestyle. (This would be the current complaint for hospitalization, a description of its onset, characteristics, and course since onset.)

The patient's perceived postdischarge needs.
Physical status including a review of systems.
Prehospitalization resource use.

Self-care practices:
- Focus on strengths and abilities intact
- Inquire about expectations and desires

Medication history:
- Dosage
- Time of administration
- Route
- Food or beverage taken with medication
- Allergies or reactions
- Discontinued drugs
- Over-the-counter medications used
- Home remedies

Nutritional history:
- Usual meal times
- Ability to feed self? Chew? Swallow?
- Prescription diets or own diet
- Food allergies or intolerances
- Religious practices related to diet
- Vitamins, food supplements, or health foods

Psychological health

Mental/emotional status:
- Cognition
- Affective state/mood
- Behavior

Social health

Family relationships:
- Health status of family members
- Patient's role in the family
- Other relationships, including pets

TABLE 3.1 *Continued*

Functional health

Activities of daily living, for example:
- Bathes and dresses self with or without functional devices
- Feeds self

Instrumental activities of daily living, for example:
- Does own shopping
- Drives own car or uses other transportation services
- Prepares meals
- Cleans own house, makes beds, etc.

The patient's typical day and habits including:
- Eating habits
- Rest and sleep patterns
- Physical and recreational activities, hobbies
- Personal hygiene practices
- Elimination patterns
- Volunteer work, clubs, organizational, and other working or religious activities
- Use of drugs or alcohol
- Social visits

Environmental health

The neighborhood:
- Density of buildings and population
- Socialization pattern of neighbors
- Access to stores, religious affiliations, clubs, etc.
- Transportation accommodations

The home:
- House, apartment, condominium
- Use of stairs, elevators, handrails
- Maintenance of yard (if house)
- Shower and tub (stepping into and out of)
- Presence of scatter rugs
- Amount of furniture
- Possessions with special meaning
- Noise levels
- Lighting
- Heating

and relates them to the discharge process. There are four main predictors of postdischarge outcomes of the hospitalized elderly that can be identified through patient assessment:

1. *The patients' perceptions of their own general health.* Patients who believe that their health is good or excellent have a much better chance of regaining health after hospitalization even with a high degree of disability present (Johnson & Fethke, 1985).

2. *The complexity of medical conditions.* Examples of variables affecting postdischarge outcome include severity of illness, presence of multiple other chronic conditions, discharge diagnosis, and medication regimen (Kane, Matthias, & Sampson, 1983). For example, an older patient with multiple chronic conditions and a complicated medication regimen is more likely to be readmitted or institutionalized than an older patient with no chronic ailments and few medications.

3. *Patients' inability to maintain responsibility for their own health.* Patients with mental status deficits, functional deficits, a history of repeated hospitalizations during the previous 12 months, and the repeated use of community agencies for health and social services prior to admission are more likely to experience poor postdischarge outcomes such as repeat hospitalizations (Berkman & Abrams, 1986; Inui, Stevenson, Plorde, & Murphy, 1981; Johnson & Fethke, 1985; Kane et al., 1983; Lamont, Sampson, Matthias, & Kane, 1983; Wolock, Schlesinger, Dinerman, & Seaton, 1987).

4. *The presence of family or social networks capable of providing needed support* (Johnson & Fethke, 1985). Patients with no informal support systems or with care needs that surpass the capabilities of their families are at risk for poor postdischarge outcomes.

PHYSICAL ASSESSMENT

Assessment of the older adult differs from that of younger adults. Structural age-related changes alter physical findings on examination and influence the manner of presentation of many disease processes. The typical signs and symptoms for a particular disease may be absent or replaced by something as vague as an acute confusional state. Prescription drugs may also affect the older adult in an uncustomary way, making assessment an even more difficult task.

Distinguishing Between the Normal Changes of Aging and the Processes of Illness

Aging is a complex, normal, and inevitable process characterized by changes in cells, tissues, and organs that effect structure and function of the older individual. Aging is not a disease. Examples of aging include menopause, lens changes in the eyes, and stiffening of the arterial walls.

Examples of disease, on the other hand, include dementia, incontinence, osteoporosis, and depression.

A clinical appreciation for the effects of normal aging on physiological and functional processes will, most likely, contribute to a decrease in morbidity and mortality in acutely ill and critically compromised elders (Walker, 1992). Four attributes of aging bear watching by the discharge team.

First, some of the progressive and irreversible changes associated with aging are harmful in and of themselves (Kohn & Monnier, 1987). For example, older individuals experience a decrease in:

- conduction velocity
- basal metabolic rate
- standard cell water
- cardiac index
- standard glomerular filtration rate (inulin)
- vital capacity
- standard renal plasma flow (diodrast)
- standard renal plasma flow (PAH)
- maximal breathing capacity

Aging and associated degenerative processes create an internal environment that predisposes older individuals to sustain further insult from exposure to chemical, functional, or physical factors to which they would otherwise be resistant (Kohn & Monnier, 1987). For example, older individuals are not only more susceptible to hip fractures—due to many age-related problems such as transient ischemic attacks, rapid drop in blood pressure, and osteoporosis—but also experience increased mortality associated with hip fracture (Riffel, 1982).

Second, the elderly are more prone to specific ailments. According to Kohn and Monnier (1987), there are certain pathologies that demonstrate an increased incidence with increasing age. The respiratory system undergoes the greatest age-related change and decrease in function; vital capacity and respiration depth decrease and the muscles of respiration weaken (diaphragm, intercostal muscles, and accessory muscles), reducing efficiency of respiration and creating less depth of inspiratory and expiratory force. Thus respiratory ailments are much more devastating for the elderly.

Third, the elderly are more likely to feel the effects of a disturbance in one system in other systems as well. Multiple pathology, the presence of more than one condition or illness, occurs more commonly in older individuals. According to Eberle and Besdine (1992), the presence of multiple pathologies may lead to an accumulation of disabilities. Accumulation of functional losses can occur as an interaction between diseases or between disease and treatments or medications (Besdine, 1988).

Fourth, the elderly present signs and symptoms of a disease atypically. For example, a myocardial infarction may be asymptomatic in an older person. Pain, if any, may be in the shoulder or jaw. There may also be a vague sense of indigestion. The first sign of a urinary tract infection in the elderly may be an acute confusional state, rather than the usual dysuria and frequency. Fever and pleuritic pain may be absent in pneumonia, with confusion and restlessness being the only symptoms. Note that acute episodes of confusion are never a normal or expected part of aging. Very often these episodes are due to reversible causes, such as infection, dehydration, or medications, and should be treated as an emergency.

A Review of Systems

The physical assessment is one of the most important steps in the discharge planning process. Before he or she can determine the patient's ability to function after discharge, the nurse must have an understanding of the effects that certain physiological changes might have on the patient's health and the multisystem failures that can occur with aging.

Appendix A provides a comprehensive list of physiological changes that occur during the normal aging process and notes the common disturbances that result from these changes. While reviewing the list, focus on the ways the major effects of aging mentioned above play out during the systems review and physical assessment of the older individual.

PSYCHOLOGICAL/MENTAL ASSESSMENT

Psychological Changes in the Later Years

Cognitive ability in old age changes only with respect to pace of information processing. In other, words older people require more time for learning. The three stages of information processing are registration, storage, and retrieval.

Registration is the act of attending to and absorbing information. The older person is affected by the environment (for example, simultaneous stimuli can be confusing), age-related sensory-perceptual changes, and the pacing of information. In the case of an elderly patient who suffered scald burns, you want to make sure that he or she is able to return to a safer home environment and is knowledgeable about precautions to take to avoid future injury. Thus, registration is very important. If the patient has shown signs of not absorbing the information, make sure to remove all distractions from the room during the talk, and deliver messages that are short and suggest actions that are easy to follow. If the patient is still unable to register, perhaps a mental status examination is necessary.

Storage of information is commonly called memory. Short-term memory has two components: primary and secondary. Primary memory represents a store of limited capacity in which contents are subject to displacement, and secondary memory represents a rehearsal-dependent store of a relatively large capacity (Waugh & Norman, 1965). Elders do more poorly in secondary (organizational properties) than primary memory tasks. However, training programs can improve secondary memory performance.

Ability to retrieve information is difficult to measure. In general, elders have been found to retrieve information more slowly from secondary memory. However, recall tests often used to determine information retrieval ability are not altogether reliable. They involve emotional reactions, such as fear of being wrong.

Morale in old age is often influenced by health and financial status. Morale is defined as the way one views, with satisfaction and happiness, one's own life and includes feelings about the past, present, and future. High morale correlates positively with good perceptions of health and financial status. A patient burdened by poor health, other than normal aging changes, and by financial strain may need help in dealing with these problems before and after being discharged.

Self-concept or self-esteem is the attitude one has about oneself. Its assessment is derived from three components: factual information about that attitude, how one feels about the attitude, and how one is motivated by the attitude (Meisenhelder, 1985). For example, patients with a very low self-concept may not be able to visualize themselves overcoming functional and physical problems. And like morale and cognitive functioning, self-concept has implications for compliance with medical and nursing regimens, as well as with the motivational capacity of patients to re-educate themselves to live with functional deficits.

Mental Status Assessment

When measuring the degree of psychological changes that occur during old age, nurses should understand that there are several factors that influence the outcome of such tests. Before administering a mental status test, carefully observe patient behavior during the health history. It may provide you with information on a patient's mental health status. Specifically, observe the patient's

- appearance, posture, and behavior
- grooming and personal hygiene
- facial expression and affect
- speech (clearness, articulation, level of vocabulary)
- coherency of thought process
- mood
- manner of relating to things in the environment

Assess cognitive function. It is particularly important to assess cognitive changes in the elderly because they may signal dementia and because eligibility for long-term care services is often linked to level of cognitive function (Mezey, Rauckhorst, & Stokes, 1993). Two commonly used measures of cognitive function include the Mini-Mental State Examination (MMSE) and the Short Portable Mental Status Questionnaire (SPMSQ).

The MMSE (Table 3.2) contains 11 questions that assess both verbal responses and performance (Folstein, Folstein, & McHugh, 1975). The test, which can be administered in about 10 minutes, differentiates between patients with delirium, dementia, and depression.

TABLE 3.2 The Mini-Mental State Exam

Patient _____ Examiner _____ Date _____

Maximum score	Score	
		Orientation
5	( )	What is the (year) (season) (date) (day) (month)?
5	( )	Where are we (state) (country) (town) (hospital) (floor)?
		Registration
3	( )	Name 3 objects: 1 second to say each. Then ask the patient all 3 after you have said them. Give 1 point for each correct answer. Then repeat them until he/she learns all 3. Count trials and record.
		Trials _____
		Attention and Calculation
5	( )	Serial 7s. 1 point for each correct answer. Stop after 5 answers. Alternatively spell "world" backward.
		Recall
3	( )	Ask for the 3 objects repeated above. Give 1 point for each correct answer.
		Language
2	( )	Name a pencil and watch. (2 points)
1	( )	Repeat the following "No, ifs, ands, or buts." (1 point)
3	( )	Follow a 3-stage command. "Take a paper in your hand, fold it in half, and put it on the floor." (3 points)
1	( )	Read and obey the following: CLOSE YOUR EYES. (1 point)
1	( )	Write a sentence. (1 point)
1	( )	Copy design. (1 point)
_____		**Total Score**
		ASSESS level of consciousness along a continuum. _____
		Alert Drowsy Stupor Coma

Note. From "Mini-mental state: A practical method for grading the cognitive state of patients for the clinician," by M.E. Folstein and S.E. Folstein, 1975, *Journal of Psychiatric Research, 12*, 189–198. Copyright Elsevier Science Ltd. Reprinted by permission.

A perfect score on the MMSE is 30. Those scoring below 21 are considered to have dementia, delirium, or depression (Folstein et al., 1975). Guidelines for administering the MMSE are included in Appendix B.

The SPMSQ (Table 3.3) scores allow for differentiation among four levels of disability. The spread of possible scores is 10, with a score of 8 or higher indicating intact cognition. Lower scores differentiate among mild, moderate, and severe cognitive impairment (see Pfeiffer, 1975).

Because a patient's performance in testing may be influenced by many socioeconomic and disease factors, administer a mental status examination more than once. Patients may be able to perform better at different points in the day when they are without pain or anxiety. An elder who is admitted in a state of obvious poor hygiene may need further evaluation and subsequent discharge planning to ensure that needs are being met. Many times the confused elder is labeled "senile" or "incompetent," when in fact the confusion could be only a temporary state. Confusion does lead to other increasingly complex problems if the underlying cause is not detected and treated.

Be aware that depression, a common occurrence in older people, may be confused with and mistakenly diagnosed as dementia or delirium. Depression or confusion, however, may be reversible by treatment. Symptoms of depression that mock dementia include:

- lack of concern about hygiene and appearance
- lack of involvement in daily activities
- decreased attention span
- tendency to withdraw
- lack of emotion

However, there are certain signs that distinguish the two. In general, demented patients exhibit gradual, progressive, deterioration, whereas those with depression have a more acute onset and the cognitive deficit is nonprogressive. Patients with depression often have a past or family history of depression. They may complain of severe memory loss, but will often perform better than expected on mental status examinations. Depressed patients often have had a recent stress that may have led to the depression.

Some patients may have both dementia and depression. Depression presenting as dementia includes:

TABLE 3.3   Short Portable Mental Status Questionnaire (SPMSQ)

Instructions: Ask questions 1 through 10 in this list and record all answers. Ask question 4A only if patient does not have a telephone. Record total number of errors based on ten questions.

+	−

1. What is the date today?_____
   Month   Day   Year

2. What day of the week is it?_____

3. What is the name of this place?_____

4. What is your telephone number?_____

4A. What is your street address?_____

   (Ask only if patient does not have a telephone.)_____

5. How old are you?_____

6. When were you born?_____

7. Who is the President of the U.S. now?_____

8. Who was the President before him?_____

9. What was your mother's maiden name?_____

10. Subtract 3 from 20 and keep subtracting 3 from each new number, all the way down.

Total Number of Errors

Scoring: 0–2 errors = intact mental function
3–4 errors = mild intellectual impairment
5–7 errors = moderate intellectual impairment
8–10 errors = severe intellectual impairment
Allow one more error if subject had only grade school education
Allow one fewer error if subject has had education beyond high school.

Note. Adapted from "A short portable mental status questionnaire for the assessment of organic brain deficit in elderly patients," by E. Pfeiffer, 1975, *Journal of the American Geriatrics Society, 23,* 433–441. Copyright American Geriatrics Society. Reprinted by permission.

- rapid onset of intellectual loss
- little or no progression of deficit
- prior history of depression
- objective testing showing better memory than patient's complaint
- recent provocative stress

Planning for discharge needs should be based upon the real ability of a patient to function in the posthospital environment. If testing yields inaccurate data then the plan will not meet the patient's real needs.

FUNCTIONAL ASSESSMENT

Because preserving functional ability is an important health objective, functional assessment is probably the most crucial component of the patient assessment.

This section looks at the functional assessment as a way of measuring a patient's ability to manage in everyday life. Functional assessment consists of two components: (a) the activities of daily living (ADLs) or the elder's ability to manage personal care and (b) the instrumental activities of daily living (IADLs) or the elder's ability to live independently in the community.

The Utility of Functional Status Measures

The functional assessment is essential to discharge planning for several reasons. First, it is useful in identifying potential disabilities and problems needing remediation. Second, it can be used to measure impaired function and self-care abilities. When assessing a patient for functional status keep in mind that hospitals provide atmospheres of dependency and patients may be able to perform activities outside of the hospital that are done for them in the institution. Nurses, however, need to make sure that they assess an actual performance of the activities, not assumed ability of the patient to perform them. Third, functional assessment is used to identify individual needs, which must be known prior to the appropriate selection of posthospital services.

One must be careful to use the results of these examinations in concert with other history and clinical findings. A low score for any particular patient does not necessarily mean institutionalization. Other factors, such as social supports, may help keep the patient in the home environment. One cannot accurately predict posthospital needs with a single administration of a test. The tests are meant to be used to measure a person's progress over time and should be administered at intervals. With these provisos, functional assessment helps determine whether long-term care services are needed.

Standardized Tools to Measure Functional Status

There are many standardized tools to measure functional status that have been developed and tested for reliability and validity and used in research studies. These tools are often used in rehabilitation and in long-term care settings. However, many acute care settings are now using some type of functional tool to measure patient needs. For example, Beth Israel Hospital in Boston, Massachusetts, uses a nursing assessment tool—Functional Health Pattern Assessment—to measure initial status. Information about patient status is then documented on a daily basis in the chart and also through a computerized system.

The tools below are all useful in determining functional capabilities of patients. However, it is important to note that setting determines, to some extent, the type of assessment tool utilized.

Marge Gordon's (1982) Functional Health Pattern Assessment (FHPA) is widely used and accepted as a valid and reliable nursing tool for gathering critical information regarding instrumental and basic activities of daily living. Because the instrument is comprehensive, gathering patient perceptions of typical day-to-day practices, it does not fit the narrow definition of a functional assessment. Yet, the inclusion of additional categories, such as mental health, contribute to its usefulness. The indices included on this tool are (a) health perception/health management, (b) metabolic/nutrition, (c) elimination, (d) activity/exercise, (e) sleep/rest, (f) cognitive/perceptual, (g) self-perception/self-concept, (h) roles/relationships, (i) sexuality/reproductive, (j) coping/stress tolerance, and (k) value/belief.

In the Gordon FHPA, functional status is measured as part of the patient's perceived ability for feeding, bathing, toileting, bed mobility, dressing, grooming, general mobility, cooking, home maintenance, and housekeeping (Gordon, 1982). The patient's perceived ability at each of these activities is then coded by the nurse as follows:

Level 0: Full self-care

Level I: Requires use of equipment or device

Level II: Requires assistance or supervision from another person

Level III: Requires assistance or supervision from another person and equipment or device

Level IV: Is dependent and does not participate (in the assessment interview)

Measures of activities of daily living (ADL) assess people's ability to manage their personal care (for example, bathing, dressing, hygiene, feeding, transferring, toileting). Three widely accepted tools are the Katz Index, the Barthel Index, and the Lawton Scale.

The Katz Index of ADL (Table 3.4) was developed over 30 years ago and is also widely used. It has been described as the functional assessment most consistently useful and carefully studied in the hospital setting. The Katz Index measures six functions—bathing, Dressing, toileting, transfer, continence, and feeding—using a dichotomous rating scale of independent/dependent among hierarchically ordered tasks (Kane & Kane, 1988).

The Katz index assumes that recovery of function progresses through three stages:

1. Early independence in feeding and continence
2. Subsequent recovery of transfer and toileting
3. Complex independence in bathing and dressing

The Barthel Index was developed in 1965. It is widely used in rehabilitation settings and in studies of stroke recovery. The Barthel includes ten ADL and differentiates for each variable between whether an activity is performed totally independently, with human aid, or with use of an assistive device, and whether the activity is performed in a reasonable amount of time (Kane & Kane, 1988). The patient is assigned a numerical score for each category, with a maximum score of 100 indicating independence. Any score less than 40 signifies severe dependence. (A score less than 60 indicates a need for long-term care 90% of the time.)

Measures of IADLs assess a range of activities more complex than personal care (Kane & Kane, 1981). Instrumental activities of daily

Table 3.4   Katz Index of ADL

Independence means without supervision, direction, or active personal assistance, except as specifically noted below. This is based on actual status and not ability. A patient who refuses to perform a function is considered as not performing the function, even though he or she is deemed able.

Bathing (sponge, shower, or tub)
Independent: assistance only in bathing a single part (back or disabled extremity) or bathes self completely
Dependent: Assistance in bathing more than one part of body; assistance in getting in or out of tub; does not bathe self

Dressing
Independent: gets clothes from closets and drawers; puts on clothes, outer garments, braces; manages fasteners; act of tying shoes is excluded
Dependent: does not dress self or remains partly undressed

Going to Toilet
Independent: gets to toilet; gets on and off toilet; arranges clothes, cleans organs of excretion (may manage own bedpan used at night only and may or may not be using mechanical supports)
Dependent: uses bedpan or commode or receives assistance in getting to and using toilet

Transfer
Independent: moves in and out of bed and in and out of chair independently (may or may not be using mechanical supports)
Dependent: assistance in moving in or out of bed and/or chair; does not perform one or more transfers

Continence
Independent: urination and defecation entirely self-controlled
Dependent: partial or total incontinence in urination or defecation; partial or total control by enemas, catheters, or regulated use of urinals and/or bedpans

Feeding
Independent: gets food from plate or its equivalent into mouth (precutting of meat and preparation of food, such as buttering bread, are excluded from evaluation)
Dependent: assistance in act of feeding; does not eat at all or parenteral feeding

Evaluation Form

Name _____   Date of Evaluation _____

For each area of functioning listed below, circle description that applies (the word "assistance" means supervision, direction, or personal assistance).

Bathing—either sponge bath, tub bath, or shower

Receives no assistance (gets in and out of tub by self if tub is usual means of bathing)	Receives assistance in bathing only one part of body (such as back or a leg)	Receives assistance in bathing more than one part of body (or does not bathe self)

Dressing—gets clothes from closets and drawers; puts on clothes, including underclothes, outer garments; manages fasteners (including braces, if worn)

Gets clothes and gets completely dressed without assistance	Gets clothes and gets dressed without assistance except for tying shoes	Receives assistance in getting clothes or in getting dressed or stays partly or completely undressed

Toileting—going to the "toilet room" for bowel and urine elimination; cleaning self after elimination and arranging clothes

Goes to "toilet room," cleans self, and arranges clothes without assistance (may use object for support such as cane, walker, or wheelchair and may manage night bedpan or commode, emptying same in morning)	Receives assistance in going to "toilet room" or in cleansing self or in arranging clothes after elimination or in use of night bedpan or commode	Does not go to room termed "toilet" for the elimination process

Transfer

Moves in and out of bed and in and out of chair without assistance (may use object for support such as cane or walker)	Moves in or out of bed or chair with assistance	Does not get out of bed

Continence

Controls urination and bowel movement completely by self	Has occasional "accidents"	Supervision helps keep urine or bowel control; catheter is used or is incontinent

Feeding

Feeds self without assistance	Feeds self except for getting assistance cutting meat or buttering bread	Receives assistance in feeding or is fed partly or completely by tubes or intravenous fluids

Note. From "Studies of illness in the aged. The index of ADL: A standardized measure of biological and psychosocial function," by S. Katz, A. B. Ford, R. S. Moskowitz, B. A. Jackson, and M. W. Jackson, 1963, *Journal of the American Medical Association*, 185, 94–98. Copyright American Medical Association. Reprinted by permission.

TABLE 3.5 Scale for Instrumental Activities of Daily Living (IADL)

Male score			Female score
	A.	**Ability to use telephone**	
1		1. Operates telephone on own initiative; looks up and dials numbers, etc.	1
1		2. Dials a few well-known numbers	1
1		3. Answers telephone but does not dial	1
0		4. Does not use telephone at all	0
	B.	**Shopping**	
1		1. Takes care of all shopping needs independently	1
0		2. Shops independently for small purchases	0
0		3. Needs to be accompanied on any shopping trip	0
0		4. Completely unable to shop	0
	C.	**Food Preparation**	
		1. Plans, prepares, and serves adequate meals independently	1
		2. Prepares adequate meals if supplied with ingredients	0
		3. Heats and serves prepared meals, or prepares meals but does not maintain adequate diet	0
		4. Needs to have meals prepared and served	0
	D.	**Housekeeping**	
		1. Maintains house alone or with occasional assistance (e.g., heavy-work domestic help)	1
		2. Performs light daily tasks such as dishwashing and bed making	1
		3. Performs light daily tasks but cannot maintain acceptable level of cleanliness	1
		4. Needs help with all home maintenance tasks	1
		5. Does not participate in any housekeeping tasks	0
	E.	**Laundry**	
		1. Does personal laundry completely	1
		2. Launders small items; rinses socks, stockings, etc.	1
		3. All laundry must be done by others	0
	F.	**Mode of transportation**	
1		1. Travels independently on public transportation or drives own car	1
1		2. Arranges own travel via taxi, but does not otherwise use public transportation	1

TABLE 3.5 *Continued*

Male score			Female score
0	3.	Travels on public transportation when assisted or accompanied by another	1
0	4.	Travel limited to taxi or automobile, with assistance of another	0
0	5.	Does not travel at all	0
	G.	**Responsibility for own medication**	
1	1.	Is responsible for taking medication in correct dosages at correct time	1
0	2.	Takes responsibility if medication is prepared in advance in separate dosages	0
0	3.	Is not capable of dispensing own medication	0
	H.	**Ability to handle finances**	
1	1.	Manages financial matters independently (budgets, writes checks, pays rent and bills, goes to bank); collects and keeps track of income	1
	2.	Manages day-to-day purchases, but needs help with bank for major purchases, etc.	1
0	3.	Incapable of handling money	0

Note. From "Assessment of older people: Self-maintaining and instrumental activities for daily living," by H. P. Lawton and E. M. Brody, 1969, *The Gerontologist, 9,* 179. Copyright The Gerontological Society of America. Reprinted by permission.

living (e.g., cooking, laundering, managing medication, managing finances, public transportation, using the telephone) are difficult to measure in the hospital since individual abilities to live independently in the community are involved. The most commonly used measure of IADL is the Lawton IADL Scale, (Table 3.5) which differentiates as to whether the activity is performed with no, minimal, or substantial assistance, or not at all (Lawton, 1971).

HELPING THE ELDERLY ADAPT TO FUNCTIONAL CHANGES

Helping elders cope is at the crux of success in the home and community. The major difference between those elders who become institutionalized and those who remain at home lies in their ability to develop coping skills and support mechanisms.

To begin helping persons learn coping skills, the nurse should first identify the patient's image of self in relation to ability to cope. The impact of hospitalization frequently causes older persons to become more dependent and the reality is that, frequently, the elderly are more seriously impaired upon exiting the hospital than when they entered the hospital.

The Nurse's Roles

The nurse has five major roles in helping the elder learn new coping skills and adjust to changes. These include, but are not limited to, the following roles.

Facilitator of Increased Mobility and Strength

Rehabilitation for the older patient is essential. Rather than focusing on the problem-oriented approach to care, nurses should move their attention to those strengths or needs of the patient that can be addressed successfully. This approach helps increase level of functioning and decrease dependency.

Patient Advocate

Have there been situations in which you needed to or did act as an advocate for a patient? In what way did this improve the patients coping ability?

As a primary caregiver the nurse is in the ideal position to act as spokesperson for patients, especially when patients are not able to perform decision-making tasks themselves. The complexity of community services that raise issues of accessibility, eligibility, and funding requirements place the already functionally disabled elder at a disadvantage in securing and coordinating needed services. The nurse can assist the patient in applying for services and/or medical supplies and obtaining them. However, it is important to note that if the patient is able to assist in the decision-making process on any of these tasks, nurses should make sure that they involve the patient.

Educator

As an educator, the nurse identifies areas of knowledge deficits in relation to resources, finances, medication administration and interaction, safety, and nutrition. Once they determine the patient's gaps in knowledge, nurses implement educational programs to fill the gaps. Educational efforts may target family members and/ or significant others in addition to or instead of the patient directly.

Support Resource Person

One of the most frequent reasons for institutionalization is lack of informal support systems. Elders may focus inward and decrease the scope of their social interactions. In addition, losses and functional changes can reduce the number of informal support systems available. A major step toward allowing persons to remain in their home is developing a plan to ensure that daily needs are met. This can be accomplished by coordinating efforts of both formal and informal support systems such as family, friends, health care agency workers, neighbors, and volunteer services.

As a support resource person, nurses assist patients and their families in establishing a reliable informal and formal support system. The following are some ways this might be accomplished:

- Assess the family's ability to act as caregiver.
- Prepare the adult children for a shift in dependency as their parents age.
- Recognize the interrelationships, independence, and reciprocity of family members' roles.
- Support the elderly person in efforts to maintain autonomy, to participate in care and decision making.
- Establish a relationship with the family and support all family members.
- Involve family members in the care of the hospitalized or institutionalized older person if they desire.
- Help the family identify and use resources such as respite care and counseling.

- Teach family members about the normal aging process and possible physical and mental problems of elderly parents.
- Help family members negotiate the sharing of care activities
- Prepare the patient and family for changes in setting.

Facilitator of Self-Esteem

Self-esteem is the image or evaluation one has about oneself based upon acceptance by others. When self-esteem is low, the elder avoids interacting with others and does not attempt new challenges, is unable to solve problems, set goals, or take action (Norris & Kunes-Connell, 1987). Elders with poor self-images tend to isolate themselves and may become depressed.

The nurse can facilitate and enhance self-esteem in several ways: by helping patients succeed in self-care skills, thus increasing the patients' perceived control; by promoting positive statements about self and eliminating self-derogatory statements; by having patients look at their abilities and share knowledge of these abilities in interactions with others; and by helping patients modify role expectations when appropriate.

The Nurse's Solutions

Features of a physical assessment, mental status examination, and functional assessment have been described in this chapter. Using these measures, nurses can gather pertinent patient information and draw from these data to identify discharge needs. However, nurses' decisions about in-hospital care can also ensure better patient outcomes at discharge.

For the case descriptions that follow, we have developed protocols of care for patients with specific discharge needs. In these cases,* the patient is either (a) unable to prepare own meals, (b) unfamiliar with the medication regimen, (c) needing assistance bathing and dressing, or (d) susceptible to falls. Each description includes a brief patient history, including gender, age, reason for hospitalization, nursing diagnosis, behavior, living situation, personal history, needs, and resources.

---

* These cases were adapted from ones originally developed by Eileen Kitchen, RN, MS; and Marion Phipps, RN, MS.

The protocols developed for each situation name the functional impairment and identify nursing actions that can be initiated in the hospital and ones that can be followed in the community. Remember that the focus of functional assessments in the hospital and home is to identify means of adapting to impairment in order to maintain as normal a lifestyle as possible. Most elderly wish to return to their homes.

Case Study 1: *Mr. Lieberman*

Mr. Lieberman is an 83-year-old man who was admitted to the emergency department for failure to thrive. Prior to admission he lived alone and had been widowed for approximately 1 year. He was malnourished and depressed. He reported no close family except for two sons who live hours away. The superintendent of his building reported that his apartment was in disarray and that Mr. Lieberman seldom prepared his own meals.

Functional Impairment

Impaired home maintenance

Solutions

In the hospital . . .

1. Educate the patient regarding services available such as homemaker, meals-on-wheels, and congregate meals.
2. Assess support structures for help from family and friends.
3. Educate future providers about diet preferences and needs.
4. Attempt to ensure socialization features in posthospital environment meal arrangement.
5. Ask patient his or her desires and preferences for arrangements

6. Actively engage the patient in developing a plan to meet this need.

In the community . . .

1. Follow through on how meals are actually being arranged and the level of satisfaction the patient feels with the plan developed.

Case Study 2: *Mrs. Rogers*

Mrs. Rogers is an 83-year-old woman who lived alone and functioned independently prior to hospitalization. She "ruled in" for a large SEMI and has an ejection fraction of 12%. She tires easily and requires oxygen at 2L nasal prong at all times. On repeated Mini-Mental State exams, she scored 24/30 with primary deficits in recall and attention.

After discharge Mrs. Rogers will need to adhere to a medication regimen of

10 mg Nifedipine PO tid,

30 mg Diltiazem PO qid,

40 mg Lasix in AM and 20 mg in PM, and

32 mEq Kcl qd.

She did not take any medications prior to admission and requests to return home upon discharge.

Functional Impairment

Knowledge deficit

Solutions

In the hospital . . .

1. Prepare a plan for educating the patient about the medication.

2. Prepare a schedule for the patient to use at home.

3. Assess the patient for any sensory or functional deficits that may present problems in self-administration.

4. If present, develop an informal support system for administration and teach those people.

5. Inquire about other medications the patient would normally use in the home environment that may interact with the prescription drug.

6. Educate accordingly.

7. Enlist the patient's participation in developing a discharge plan for self-help at home and for monitoring any follow-up lab work needed to monitor levels of the drug.

In the community . . .

1. Ascertain knowledge and adherence to plan

Community services might include

- Transportation services to have laboratory work done
- Delivery by drugstores
- Informal supports from family and friends (if available)

Case Study 3: *Mrs. Price*

Mrs. Price is an 87-year-old woman who has lived for many years in her own apartment in an elderly housing complex. She has been independent and enjoyed shopping trips and traveling with friends. However, on a recent shopping trip, she was struck by a car while attempting to cross the street. She was brought to the hospital emergency department where she was treated for multiple fractures to her right upper extremity. Now, her right arm is in a cast and she wears a sling. Despite this, Mrs. Price asked to return home after discharge. She has difficulty performing her activities of daily living and will be dependent with bathing and dressing.

Functional Impairment

Self-care deficit: Bathing/hygiene, dressing/grooming

Solutions

In the hospital . . .

1. Ascertain level of ability to assist self.
2. Teach use of devices to assist in dressing and bathing.
3. Attempt to bring the patient to an independent level with use of equipment and other adaptations.
4. With the patient, develop a plan to adapt the home environment for independent use of tub/shower and dressing devices and/or assistance from informal or skilled support people.

In the community . . .

1. Observe hygiene and grooming.
2. Elicit compliance with the plan developed by patient and others and satisfaction of the patient with services.

Community services might include

- CHORE services to install equipment
- Home Health Aide services
- Informal supports

Case Study 4: *Mrs. Morgan*

Mrs. Morgan is a 77-year-old woman who was admitted to the hospital after a fall. She has had two previous emergency department admissions for falling in her home. Fortunately, she has not sustained any fractures or other traumas with these falls.

Mrs. Morgan has a history of Parkinson's disease, degenerative arthritis of both hips, and orthostatic hypotension. The geriatric team evaluated Mrs. Morgan and determined that her gait disorder, secondary to Parkinson's, and the postural hypotension may have caused the falls.

Functional Impairment

Impaired physical mobility

Solutions

In the hospital . . .

1. Teach the patient how to move about the home environment in order to avoid falls.
2. Assess and teach any knowledge deficit in skin care and dietary needs arising from immobility.
3. Assess prehospital environment and, with the patient, develop a plan for adaptation of home to meet needs.
4. Check reimbursement or financial assistance services for any necessary restructuring of the home environment.
5. Assess needs in other areas affected by impaired physical mobility, such as meal preparation, bathing, shopping, housekeeping, and laundry.
6. Ascertain and/or help arrange informal supports.

In the community . . .

1. Evaluate home arrangement of rooms and bathroom accessibility.
2. Ascertain satisfaction with arrangements and use of any support systems.

Community services might include

- Volunteer services
- CHORE services
- Homemaker services
- Home health aides

SUMMARY

The key points of the chapter are:

1. Determinants of patient outcomes at discharge include patients' perception of health, the complexity of medical conditions, the patients' ability to maintain responsibility for their health, and the presence of family and social networks who can provide support.

2. Physical assessment of the older adult differs from that of younger adults. Structural, age-related changes alter physical findings on examination and influence the manner of presentation of many disease processes. Typical signs and symptoms for a particular disease may be absent or replaced by something as vague as an acute confusional state. Medications may affect older adults in an unusual way.

3. Although most elderly benefit from treatment provided in the hospital, many elderly patients experience adverse events during and following hospitalization.

4. It is particularly important to assess cognitive changes in the elderly because they may signal dementia.

5. Because functional ability is closely related to the overall wellbeing of the elderly, it is important for the nurse to attend to the functional status of the elderly in the hospital.

6. Functional assessment is essential to discharge planning because it is useful in identifying potential disabilities and remediable problems, measuring impaired function and self-care abilities, and identifying individual needs prior to selection of posthospital services.

7. In order to reduce dependency resulting from hospitalization or from decreasing functional ability, nurses need to help the elderly learn to cope with their inabilities by focusing on their abilities and resources.

CLINICAL EXERCISES

1. Monitor admission for one week for all patients over 65 years on your unit and list in writing five admitting diagnoses that appear to be high-risk indicators for institutionalization and/or rehospitalization. Explain the rationale for your selections.

2. Perform a mental status assessment of a patient in your care using the Mini-Mental State Exam.
3. Perform a functional assessment of a patient in your care using one of the instruments discussed in this chapter.

REFERENCES

Berkman, B., & Abrams, R. D. (1986). Factors related to hospital readmission of elderly cardiac patients. *Social Work, 31,* 99–103.

Besdine, R. W. (1988). Functional assessment. In J. W. Rowe, & R. W. Besdine (Eds.), *Geriatric medicine* (2nd ed.) (pp. 37–51). Boston: Little, Brown.

Eberle, C. M., & Besdine, R. W. (1992). Disease in old age. In T. T. Fulmer, & M. K. Walker (Eds.), *Critical care nursing of the elderly* (pp. 48–60). New York: Springer Publishing Co.

Folstein, M. R., Folstein, S. E., & McHugh, P. (1975). Mini-mental state: A practical method for grading the cognitive state of patients for the clinician. *Journal of Psychiatric Research, 12,* 189–198.

Gordon, M. (1982). *Manual of nursing diagnosis.* New York: McGraw-Hill.

Inui, T., Stevenson, K., Plorde, D., & Murphy, I. (1981). Identifying hospital patients who need elderly discharge planning for special dispositions: A comparison of alternative techniques. *Medical Care, 19,* 922–929.

Johnson, N., & Fethke, C. (1985). Post-discharge outcomes and care planning for the hospitalized elderly. In E. McClelland, K. Kelly, & K. Buckwater (Eds.), *Continuity of care: Advancing the concept of discharge planning* (pp. 229–240). New York: Grune and Stratton.

Kane, R., & Kane, R. A. (1981). *Assessing the elderly: Apractical guide to measurement.* Lexington, MA: Lexington.

Kane, R. A., & Kane, R. L. (1988). *Assessing the elderly: A practical guide to measurement.* Lexington, MA: Lexington.

Kane, R. L., Matthias, R., & Sampson, S. (1983). The risk of nursing-home placement after acute hospitalization. *Medical Care, 21,* 1055.

Kohn, R. R., & Monnier, B. M. (1987). Normal aging and its parameters. In C. G. Swift (Ed.), *Clinical pharmacology in the elderly* (pp. 3–30). New York: Marcel Dekker.

Lamont, C. T., Sampson, S., Matthias, R., & Kane, R. (1983). The outcome of hospitalization for acute illness in the elderly. *Journal of the American Geriatrics Society, 31,* 282.

Lawton, M. P. (1971). The functional assessment of elderly people. *Journal of the American Geriatrics Society, 9,* 465–481.

Meisenhelder, J. B. (1985). Self-esteem: A closer look at clinical interventions. *International Journal of Nursing Studies, 22,* 127–135.

Mezey, M. D., Rauckhorst, L., & Stokes, S. A. (1993). *Health assessment of the older individual.* New York: Springer Publishing Co.

Naylor, M., Brooten, D., Jones, R., Lavizzo-Mourey, R., Mezey, M., & Pauly, M. (1994). Comprehensive discharge planning for the hospitalized elderly. *Annals of Internal Medicine, 120,* 999–1006.

Naylor, M. (1992). Discharge planning for hospitalized elderly. In T. T. Fulmer, & M. K. Walker (Eds.), *Critical care nursing of the elderly* (pp. 331–344). New York: Springer Publishing Co.

Norris, J., & Kunes-Connell, M. (1987). Self esteem disturbance: A clinical validation study. In A. McLane (Ed.), *Classification of nursing diagnosis.* St. Louis: C.V. Mosby.

Pfeiffer, E. (1975). A short portable mental status questionnaire for the assessment of organic brain deficit in elderly patients. *Journal of the American Geriatrics Society, 23,* 433–441.

Riffel, K. (1982). Falls: Kinds, causes, and prevention. *Geriatric Nursing, 3,* 165–169.

Walker, M. K. (1992). The physiology of normal aging: Implications for nursing management of critically compromised adults. In T. T. Fulmer, & M. K. Walker (Eds.), *Critical care nursing of the elderly* (pp. 32–47). New York: Springer.

Waugh, N. C., & Norman, D. (1965). Primary memory. *Psychological Review, 72,* 89–104.

Wolock, I., Schlesinger, E., Dinerman, M., & Seaton, R. (1987). The post-hospital needs and care of patients: Implications for discharge planning. *Social Work in Health Care, 12*(4), 61–67.

SUGGESTED READINGS

Appelgate, W. B., Blass, J., & Franklin, T. (1990). Instruments for the functional assessment of older patients. *The New England Journal of Medicine, 322,* 1207–1214.

Burke, M., & Walsh, M. (1992). *Gerontological nursing: Care of the frail elderly.* St. Louis: Mosby.

Chenitz, W. C., Stone, J., & Salisbury, S. (1991). *Clinical gerontological nursing: A guide to advanced practice.* Philadelphia: Saunders.

Eliopoulos, C. (1990). *Health assessment of the older adult* (2nd ed.). Redwood City, CA: Addison-Wesley.

Lueckenotte, A. (1990). *Pocket guide to gerontologic assessment.* St. Louis: Mosby.

Mezey, M. D., Rauckhorst, L. H., & Stokes, S. A. (1993). *Health assessment of the older individual.* New York: Springer.

Resnick, N. M., Yalla, S. V., & Laureno, E. (1989). The pathophysiology of urinary incontinence among institutionalized elderly persons. *New England Journal of Medicine, 320,* 1–7.

Thomas, A. M., & Morse, J. M. (1991). Managing urinary incontinence with self-care practices. *Journal of Gerontological Nursing, 17*(6), 9–14.

APPENDIX A: Physiological Changes that Occur During the Normal Aging Process

The Five Senses

Vision
- Increased sensitivity to glare
- Decreased visual acuity, peripheral, and color vision
- Longer adjustment time for changes in lighting intensity required

Disturbances: glaucoma, cataracts

Hearing
- Loss of high-frequency tones
- Difficulty discriminating sounds when there is more than one sound

Disturbances: presbycusis (hearing loss), impacted cerumen

Smell
- Decline in acuity

Taste/oral
- Decrease in number of taste buds
- Decrease in production of saliva
- Shrinkage of the gums
- Teeth become worn

Disturbances: periodontal disease, poor nutrition

Touch

Sensory receptors are located in the skin, muscles, tendons, joints, and viscera. Important for the elderly are the sensations of heat, pain, and touch. Brain lesions or surgery and drugs may decrease or abolish the effective response to these sensations. It is important to monitor confused or demented patients.

Integument
- Wrinkling from loss of subcutaneous fat and elasticity

- Decrease in the number and activity of sweat glands
- Increasingly fragile blood supply to skin and capillaries because of loss of supporting subcutaneous fat
- Hair thins, nails thicken

Disturbances: Decubitus ulcers, stasis ulcers

Musculoskeletal System

- Skeletal muscles atrophy, strength and size decrease
- Less joint mobility
- Decreased number of muscle cells and elastic tissue
- Cartilage tissue thins
- Decreased and demineralized bone mass

Disturbances: osteoporosis, osteoarthritis, rheumatoid arthritis, hip fractures

Genitourinary System

Kidneys

- Decrease in size
- Lose ability to concentrate urine (are prone to salt depletion, dehydration, water intoxication, and excess potassium)
- Adequacy of function affected by circulatory, nervous, and endocrine systems
- Higher threshold for glucose causing hyperglycemic conditions
- Decreased ability to concentrate, dilute, and excrete drugs
- Diurnal rhythm changes (elder has to void at night)

Ureters

- May be prone to obstruction and reflux of urine

Bladder
- Smooth muscle and elastic tissue become fibrous
- Muscle tone weakens
- Bladder may fail to empty completely
- Bladder capacity is reduced
- Decreased force of stream
- Frequency of urination increases
- Bladder outlet problems: obstruction in the male, incontinence in the female
- Stretching of the bladder may cause urinary retention or urgency incontinence

Urethra
- More difficulty in opening and closing, may have increased difficulty starting a stream
- Female problems possibly due to decreased estrogen production and weakened pelvic musculature
- Male problems sometimes due to benign pro-static hypertrophy

Vagina
- Tissue atrophy from estrogen deficiency, secretions diminish, pH rises

External genitalia
- Labia atrophy from estrogen and progesterone deficiency
- Alteration in blood flow to the penis may occur

Disturbances: incontinence, urinary tract infections, benign prostatic hypertrophy, atrophic vaginitis, vaginal prolapse

Other pertinent information: Incontinence may be due to a variety of factors and is not a normal development of aging. Causes include: weakness of the muscles, inability of the kidneys to concentrate urine, side effects of medications, mechanical obstruction such as enlarged prostrate, physical immobility to get to the bathroom, dehydration (causing confusion), urinary tract infection, and most commonly, fecal impaction. Some studies have found that urinary tract infection is the most common cause of fever in elderly persons.

Gastrointestinal System

Oral cavity
- Decrease in dentine production
- Dryness of the mouth
- Oral function usually is minimally affected

Esophagus
- Does not change with age

Stomach
- Decrease in gastric mucosa with decrease in hydrochloric acid secretion
- Emptying time is prolonged

Small intestine
- Decreased height and breadth decrease surface for absorption
- Decreased absorption of nutrients

Large intestine
- Increased tortuosity
- Decreased motility and peristalsis

Pancreas
- Decreased production of lipase: leading to abnormalities of fat absorption

Liver
- Decrease in liver size and function
- Protein synthesis is reduced
- Changes in enzymes of metabolism (drug detoxification)

Gallbladder
- Decrease in emptying time of the gallbladder

Potential disturbances: xerostomia (dryness of the oral mucosa), hiatal hernia, diverticulosis, gallbladder disease, constipation/fecal impaction

Other pertinent information: Anticholinergics and anti-depressants will further increase dryness of the mouth.

Respiratory System (Undergoes the greatest age-related change and decrease in function)

- Thorax shortens and the anterior-posterior diameter increases (as in emphysema)
- Muscle tone and stretch of the chest wall decreases
- Rib cage stiffens and loses mobility because of osteoporosis and calcification of the costal cartilages
- Cilia have decreased action
- Bronchioles dilate
- Number of alveoli remains the same, but alveoli become thin and distended decreasing available surface areas for exchange of carbon dioxide and oxygen
- Reduced effectiveness of the cough and cough reflex
- Decreased vital capacity
- Reduced depth of respiration
- Weakened muscles of respiration (diaphragm, intercostal muscles, and accessory muscles) reduce efficiency of respiration and depth of inspiratory and expiratory force

Tidal volume (amount of air moved in and out with a normal breath) and respiratory rate, is relatively unchanged. Total lung volume may remain unchanged, but subcomponents of lung volume do change. Residual volume (the amount of air left in the lung after a maximal expiration) increases, thus decreasing the lung's vital capacity (less air is able to enter with the next inspiration).

The elderly compensate for these changes by relying more on the muscles of respiration, inspiration, and expiration. Conditions affecting these muscles will impact on respiratory adequacy. For example, increased intraabdominal pressure from heavy meals or body position will interfere with movement of the diaphragm.

Disturbances: pneumonia, emphysema, influenza. 1975 Census Bureau cited influenza and pneumonia jointly as the fourth leading cause of death among older persons.

Other pertinent information: Measurement of vital capacity has been cited as the most accurate predictor of the general health of an older person. Fever and pleuritic pain may be absent in pneumonia with confusion and restlessness as the only symptoms.

Cardiovascular System

- Heart muscle more stiff and less compliant
- Heart valves thicken
- Aorta less elastic, enlarged, and elongated
- Coronary circulation decreases
- Systolic B/P rises (to age of 64) then decreases
- Heart returns to its resting state more slowly after exercise
- Heart rates over 120/minute are poorly tolerated
- Number of pacemaker cells in the SA node decreases

- EKG changes: longer PR and QT intervals and changes in amplitude
- Contraction and relaxation time of the left ventricle is prolonged
- Resting heart rate remains unchanged
- Maximal heart rate, cardiac output, stroke volume, and maximal oxygen consumption all decrease
- Blood flow to organs is reduced

In general the heart should still be able to function adequately in the absence of pathology, especially during resting states, but it does require more time to adjust to stress situations.

Disturbances: myocardial infarction, congestive heart failure, hypertension, angina, lenegre's disease (microscopic lesions in the bundle branches of the conduction system causing fainting, loss of consciousness, and seizures), anemias

Other pertinent information: A myocardial infarction may be asymptomatic in an older person. Pain, if any, may be in the shoulder or jaw. There may be a vague sense of indigestion.

Mental confusion, insomnia, wandering about during the night, peripheral and presacral edema, hacking cough, distended neck veins, rapid weight gain, and the presence of a third heart sound are the signs of congestive heart failure.

Frequent awakening with a dull headache, impaired memory, and epistaxis may indicate hypertension.

Subjective symptoms of angina are decreased in older people. There may only be a vague discomfort occurring after eating.

Anemias may be caused by insidious blood loss such as that from hemorrhoids or long-term aspirin use, or from poor nutrition. Factors contributing to poor nutrition in the elderly include ill-fitting dentures, dislike of eating alone, impaired mobility to shop or cook, lack of money to buy nutritious foods, and depression. Iron deficiency anemia is the most common anemia in the elderly.

Endocrine System

- Hormone secretions decrease
- Tissue response to hormones decreases
- Glucose tolerance decreases
- Repair of tissue damage slows
- Production of antibodies and lymphocytes decreases, increasing susceptibility to disease

Disturbances: diabetes mellitus, hypothyroidism, hyperthyroidism

Other pertinent information: Behavior disorders, confusion, nocturnal headache, and slurred speech may be the first signs and symptoms of diabetes.

Neurological System

- The brain decreases in size and weight
- In the brain and spinal column the number of neurons decreases. Neurons are the basic unit for conduction nerve impulses from one part of the body to another.
- Neuroglia (supporting structure for neurons) increases
- Dendrites atrophy, producing impairment in synaptic connection and diminished electrochemical reaction (Dendrite transmission is associated with intellectual responsiveness, abstract reasoning, perception, integra-

tion of sensory input, short-term memory, and learning ability.)

- Neurotransmitter synthesis andtransmission decreases (slowed reflexes): acetylcholine, dopamine, norepinephrine, serotonin

Disturbances: Cardiovascular accident, Parkinson's disease, Alzheimer's disease, multi-infarct dementia

Other pertinent information: These changes do not necessarily affect thinking and cognition, although there is a decreased ability to respond to multiple stimuli. Implications for the nurse are to provide clear information simply and provide longer time for responses.

Loss of neurons, slowed conduction of nerve impulses, and loss of peripheral nerve functions all affect the efficiency of the system. Recovery from stress is prolonged and incomplete. Factors such as heat, cold, and extreme exercise can be harmful.

Stroke is the third leading cause of death in the elderly.

Acute episodes of confusion are never a normal or expected part of aging. Very often these episodes are due to reversible causes such as infection, dehydration, medications, etc. and should be treated as an emergency.

A gradual, progressive onset of confusion with deterioration of intellect, personality changes, and inability to carry out activities are more likely due to irreversible organic brain diseases such as Alzheimer's disease.

* Note: Appendix A was developed by Catherine Reilly-Morencif, BSN, MS, Beth Israel Hospital, Boston, MA.

APPENDIX B: Directions For Completing The Mini-Mental State Exam

All mental status examinations should be administered using the same general techniques. The methodology and areas described below coincide with the Mini-Mental State Test.

In general, begin a mental status examination only after all physiological needs of the patient have been met. The patient should be pain free, comfortable, and able to hear and see easily.

Orientation

Loss of orientation progresses from loss of time, then to place, to others, and finally to self.

- When checking for orientation, ask the patient the date, month, day, year, and season.
- Ask the patient to tell you where he or she is, and also the town, state, and country.
- If the patient does not answer completely, then specifically ask for those parts that were omitted, for example, "Can you also tell me what season it is?"
- Score 1 point for each correct answer.

Registration

Registration tests whether the patient is able to pay attention to the examiner and attend to the questions put to him or her.

- Ask the patient if you may give a memory test.
- Say the names of three unrelated objects clearly and slowly, allotting about 1 second for each one.
- After you have said all three, ask the patient to repeat them.
- Give a score of 0 to 3.
- Keep saying the names until the patient can repeat them. Allow the patient 6 trials. If he or she does not eventually learn all three items, then recall cannot be meaningfully tested.

Attention and Calculation

- Ask the patient to begin with 100 and count backwards by 7.
- Stop after five subtractions. Score the total number of correct answers.
- If the patient cannot or will not perform this counting task, ask him or her to spell the word *world* backwards. The score is the number of letters in correct order; that is, d-l-r-o-w = 5, d-l-o-r-w = 3. But if the patient will attempt even a single subtraction, score the serial 7s in preference to the spelling task.

Recall

- Ask the patient if he or she can recall the three words you previously asked him to remember. Score 0–3.

Language

- *Naming*: Show the patient a wrist watch and ask what it is. Repeat the same procedure using a pencil. Score 0–2.
- *Repetition*: Ask the patient to repeat the phrase "No ifs, ands, or buts." Score 1 point for each part correctly executed.
- *3-stage*: Give the patient a plain blank "command" piece of paper. Tell the patient to take the paper in the right hand, fold the paper in half and put it on the floor. Score 1 point for each part correctly executed.
- *Reading*: On a blank piece of paper print the sentence *Close your eyes* in letters large enough for the patient to see clearly. Ask him/her to read it and do what it says. Score 1 point only if the patient actually closes eyes.
- *Writing*: Give the patient a blank piece of paper and ask him or her to write a sentence for you. Do not dictate a sentence; it is to be written spontaneously. It must contain a subject and verb and be sensible. Correct grammar and punctuation are not necessary. Score 1 point.
- *Copying*: On a clean piece of paper, draw intersecting pentagons, each side about 2 to 5 cm. Ask the patient to copy it exactly as it is. All ten angles must be present and four lines must intersect as in the example. Ignore a tremor or rotation of the hand. Score 1 point.

Level of Consciousness

Assess level of consciousness along a continuum:

ALERT → DROWSY → STUPOR → COMA

Ascertaining level of consciousness is important for distinguishing dementia from delirium. A demented patient does not have an altered level of consciousness, whereas a delirious patient does. This difference is not important for scoring results. However, before assessing any patient be sure that he/she is aroused to the fullest and is functioning at his or her best.

The criteria for assessing level of consciousness are defined as follows:

- *Alert*: Awake. Quick. Responses are normal to tactile, verbal, and painful stimuli.

- *Drowsy*: Lethargic. Sleepy. Can be aroused to alertness with stimuli but falls asleep again easily. Yawns frequently. Falls asleep during meals and long conversations.

- *Stupor*: Totally indifferent to the environment. Vigorous stimulation is required to arouse the patient. When aroused, will attempt to defend self with purposeful movements. When aroused is slow, confused, disoriented, and may become agitated. May hallucinate.

- *Coma*: Absence of voluntary responses to any stimuli. Involuntary reflexes are present.

Interpreting the Results of the Mini-Mental State Test

One must be cautious in interpreting the results of the mini-mental state test. Socioeconomic studies have shown that level of education can greatly impact on the score results. A person with a college level education may be able to score in the "normal" range and yet still have diminished cognitive function. A person who scores within the normal range may still require further assessment for cognitive deficits. A person who scores below the normal range may not have any deficits in cognitive function, but may score low because of any number of educational, sociological, or economical factors.

Scoring Results of the Mini-Mental State

30	perfect
over 23	within a "normal" range
20–23	modest impairment
16–20	moderate impairment
below 16	severe impairment

In general, results of mental status examinations should always be reviewed in concert with findings from the patient history, physical examination, and laboratory studies.

* Adapted from "Mini-mental state: A practical method for grading the cognitive state of patients for the clinician," by M.E. Folstein and S.E. Folstein, 1975, *Journal of Psychiatric Research, 12,* 189–198.

Chapter 4

CAREGIVER ASSESSMENT

LEARNING OBJECTIVES

At the end of the chapter, readers will be able to:

1. Describe patterns of intergenerational support and provide a portrait of family care in the United States
2. Define essential components of the primary caregiver role
3. Identify the primary caregiver for elderly patients in need of support
4. Assess family dynamics, resources, and supports needed in order to help families provide adequate care to discharged patients
5. Design family interventions to reduce caregiver stress, reduce incidents of abuse and neglect, and improve the quality of family-provided care
6. Help patients and families assess what other informal sources of support they have available and utilize other informal supports, including neighbors, peers, etc., as well as formal services provided by the community

Seventy-five percent of the noninstitutionalized elderly live in family settings (Staab & Lyler, 1990). Most of these older individuals are able to function at home with the help of various family members, friends, and a variety of support services, often despite serious illness (Mezey, Rauckhorst, & Stokes, 1993). This chapter focuses specifically on those families and friends—the unpaid relatives and significant others who provide most of the ongoing, day-to-day assistance to the impaired elderly.

The chapter begins with a discussion that outlines some of the issues associated with caregiving in the United States, describing caregiving patterns, the role of caregiving in delaying institutionalization, and caregiver stress. Next, attention turns to the problems of abuse and neglect. Four cases are provided for evaluation of both the caregiving situation and the caregiving relationship. An important point to keep in mind throughout this chapter is that in each case a caregiving system is involved. Usually this system is composed of a primary dyadic relationship (primary caregiver and impaired elder) that is sometimes complemented by other informal and formal support services. If the quality of care needs to be improved, it is the system, and not just the care recipient, that must be assessed before constructive changes can be made.

It is fundamental to recognize that there is no one right way to provide care to elderly relatives who need assistance. Many caregiving options are available, utilizing a combination of informal and formal resources. Families must find a caregiving solution that works for them. The needs and capacities of both elderly relatives and of caregivers are apt to change over time; caregiving decisions need to be made and remade as circumstances change.

Because so many elderly will ultimately be discharged home to the care of family, it is important for nurses to have a better understanding of the caregiver's needs and abilities prior to discharge. Winger, Hubbard and Campbell (1992) recommend obtaining a basic data base on the family to which additional information can be added as nurses continue to interact with the family. General areas for assessment include (Kleeman, 1988):

- A realistic perception of the event by the family: for example, what is the family's understanding of the illness? What does the illness mean to the caregiver? What are his or her expectations?
- Family coping mechanisms: for example, how has the family coped in the past with similar situations? Is there anything specific about the family member's illness that would influence the caregiver's normal coping mechanisms?
- Family situational supports: for example, who is in the family? Where do the other family members live? What family members or others can be sources of support to the caregiver? Who is most affected by this illness? How? What type of support can

the caregiver or other family members provide (emotional, financial, physical care)?

FAMILY CAREGIVING

The Frail Elderly

What does it mean to be a frail elder? *Frailty*, as if applies to elderly persons, can be defined from several viewpoints. If can refer to chronological age, generally 85 and older. In the United States, there are increasing numbers of people over 85, who are sometimes called the "old-old." This means that increasing numbers of patients discharged from acute care hospitals to home are old-old. Frailty can also be defined by functional disability. For example, elderly individuals who are unable to manage the basic and/or instrumental activities of daily living are often referred to as "frail." It is necessary to consider both age and functional assessment when determining the level and type of care services the elderly will require when discharged.

When the elderly need long-term care, they turn overwhelmingly to family. Four out of five elders who are functionally impaired live in the community and rely on family, friends, and neighbors for help with one or more of their activities of daily living (ADLs) (U. S. House of Representatives, Subcommittee on Human Services of the Select Committee on Aging, 1987).

According to gerontologist Elaine Brody (1985, p 21.), the family, not the formal system, provides

> 80% to 90% of medically related and personal care, household tasks, transportation, and shopping. The family links the [elderly] to the formal support system. The family responds in emergencies and provides intermittent acute care. The family shares its home with severely impaired old people who live in the community . . . It is the dependable family that provides the expressive support—the socialization, concern, affection, and sense of having someone on whom to rely—that is the form of family help most wanted by the old.

Caregiving Patterns

A caregiving pattern is a method of delivering care. It is comprised of both those who provide care and the mechanism by which they assume that role. There are five common caregiver patterns:

1. *The chosen one* is often a primary caregiver designated by the elderly care recipient or selected by the family as the member best suited to the task. A family member may either volunteer or fall into the role of caregiver. In most cases, this person is female, typically the care recipient's wife or daughter, although sons are sometimes selected.

2. *The in-law caregiver:* If the elderly person has a son nearby but no living spouse and no daughter in close proximity, caregiving responsibility often falls not on the son but on the son's wife. The daughter-in-law may become the caregiver regardless of whether her relationship with her in-laws is good or bad; the decision can be loving and mutual or angry and forced.

3. *The caregiving team* entails any combination of family members and significant others. If there is a primary caregiver, other members of the family, as well as friends and neighbors, often provide important secondary support. These secondary caregivers become responsible for some tasks or provide "respite care" (filling in for the caregiver) so that the primary caregiver can have a break. Secondary caregivers help in other ways, too, such as participating in the decision-making process and providing emotional support to both care recipient and caregiver. In some families, the caregiving roles and responsibilities are shared and there is no single, primary caregiver.

4. *Supervised caregiving:* Some people do not provide direct care to their relatives but assume much of the responsibility for making sure that their relatives' needs are met by other people and services. Some people supervise their relatives' needs from a distance: finding services, maintaining phone contact with relatives and service providers, and visiting their relatives when they can. This can be an early stage of caregiving and also a later stage, when hiring of persons or services is more comprehensive.

5. *System caregiving:* If families are made aware of the range of possible caregiving options that exist, both informal and formal, they can utilize various combinations to form a system that supports the elder person, doesn't overwhelm any individual caregiver with responsibility, and enables the elder person to maintain as much control over his or her life as possible. Families also need to know that the pattern of care can change as the elder's needs change: What works well at one stage may not suffice when there are changes in either the elder's needs or the caregiver's ability to provide care.

Caregiver–Elder Dyad

In 1982, over 600 families who were providing care for frail elders in their homes participated in a study commissioned by the U.S. Administration on Aging and conducted by the Benjamin Rose Institute (Noelker & Poulshock, 1982). Findings from this study revealed that most care was provided by one primary caregiver. About half of the sample (305) consisted of an elder spouse caring for an elder spouse, and the other half (309) consisted of an adult child caring for the elder either alone or with spouse and children present. The emotional relationship between primary caregiver and elder proved to be the most powerful force in the caregiving situation. The study also found that about nine out of ten adult children who provided care were women; most were daughters of the elder requiring care, the rest were daughters-in-law.

The caregiver–elder dyadic relationship often becomes a powerful emotional bond, and the health of that relationship can have a major impact on the quality of care the elder receives.

Living Arrangements

The elderly consistently express a strong preference for separate living and tend to live near but separately from their children (U. S. House of Representatives, Subcommittee on Human Services of the Select Committee on Aging, 1987).

For many functionally dependent elders the necessary choice is living with relatives. When the elderly person becomes functionally dependent, shared living predominates: about 75% of all caregivers have a disabled family member or friend living with them. The decision to live together appears to be based on the aged person's need for care: one-third of the sons and 38% of the daughters, who are living with and caring for their aging and often disabled parents, said they would not have their parents live with them if the care were not needed (U.S. House of Representatives, Select Committee on Aging, 1987).

The Role of the Caregiver in Delaying Institutionalization

Family care is one of the most critical factors in preventing or delaying nursing home utilization. A study conducted by Colerick and George

(1986) examined predictors of the decision by caregivers to institution-alize elderly family members who suffer from Alzheimer's disease. It found that the single most important difference between groups of institutionalized and noninstitutionalized elders was the families' ability to care for the elders as long as necessary. As the authors explain:

> When physicians assess a patient's need for nursing home care, it is not enough to evaluate symptoms or to know how long the patient has been ill or functioning at the current cognitive level. The struc-ture and characteristics of the caregiver support system are also important, and, in fact, are better predictors of institutional place-ment than are patient characteristics. (p. 497)

The Myth of Role Reversal

Sometimes adult children who are caring for aging parents feel that roles have been reversed: When their parents start to become depen-dent on them, they then act as parents to their parents. In reality, parents never cease being parents, even when they depend on their children for many of the necessities of life.

Establishing the concept of filial maturity should be a goal. This requires that the child relate not as a parent to the elder, but as an adult child to the elderly parent. They can set proper limits and give real help without feeling overwhelmed. The result will be a more workable and rewarding relationship between the adult child and his or her parents.

Rewards and Stresses of Caregiving

Brody (1985) suggests that caregiving—having a dependent elderly parent—is becoming a normative experience for individuals and fami-lies in the United States. As a member of the caregiving system, re-member that each person in the dyad has needs, and each person also wants certain things (e.g., an elder may need to depend on others but want to be self-sufficient). A successful caregiving relationship de-pends on finding a balance between stresses and rewards.

The following quote illustrates the problems of caregiver role fatigue:

The development of role fatigue is usually gradual. Most caretakers begin by simply adding caretaking duties to their previous array of roles and responsibilities. Over time, however, two sets of interrelated things often happen. . . . Among most chronically impaired patients, health status and disabilities tend not to improve but, gradually or suddenly, to worsen, and the patient becomes increasingly dependent. At the same time, the caretaker—especially when there is only one—often becomes almost as housebound as the patient: all other roles and functions become subordinate as functions related to caretaking increasingly demand the caretaker's time and energy. (Goldstein, Regnery, & Wellin, 1981, p. 26.)

The Emotional Tug of War

There are positive and negative emotions that may come with caring for an elderly parent or spouse. Some of the positive emotions that caregivers experience might include love, compassion, tenderness, sadness, and respect. Silverstone and Hyman (1976) suggest that: when some or all of these feelings are present and are not complicated by conflicting feelings, they serve as a vital source of support and strength for both caregiver and older adult. Sometimes, however, one emotion may exist without the others. If a son respects a parent without feeling much love, his indifference may cause him pain, but he can't change it. He can still feel responsible for his parents' welfare and develop a good helping relationship.

Negative emotions that caregivers experience might include fear, anxiety, anger, and shame. Silverstone and Hyman (1976) examine these emotions further, seeking their roots.

Shame, they find, is often triggered by caregivers' feeling that they can never do enough. Adult children may also harbor fears about their parents that recall earlier days. It is common for caregivers to feel a wide range of feelings about the same person.

What other pressures might caregivers experience? Consider the following (U. S. House of Representatives, Subcommittee on Human Services of the Select Committee on Aging, 1986):

- *Outside economic pressures.* Because hospitals are under economic pressure to reduce hospitalization and to release patients more quickly into the community, pressure on the family and community to provide care increases.

- *The sandwich generation.* Many caregivers are employed and provide care and economic support to children as well as elderly relatives, a situation that has caused them to be labeled *the sandwich generation.* They must deal with competing roles and responsibilities.
- *Divorce.* Divorce can alter the family's ability to provide care.
- *Geographic dispersion.* Sharing caregiving responsibilities among family members can be hard to accomplish when some or all of the relatives live far away from the impaired elder.
- *Elderly caregivers.* As people live longer, older individuals—who may have health problems themselves—are caring for elderly spouses and maybe even older parents.
- *Federal budget controls.* The availability of formal care services has decreased in recent years in an effort to address the federal budget deficit; denial of Medicare benefits has increased.

ABUSE AND NEGLECT OF THE ELDERLY

Defining Abuse and Neglect

How do you distinguish between abuse and neglect? Consider definitions contained in state mandatory elder abuse legislation (which are abstract in nature) versus operational or measurable definitions useful in clinical situations. For example, Massachusetts General Laws (1995, p. 1) defines elder abuse as "an act or omission which results in serious physical or emotional injury to an elderly person or financial exploitation of an elderly person."

To date, all but eight states have an in-home adult abuse reporting law. Most of these laws stipulate age 60 or 65 and older as the group for which the law applies, while some adult abuse laws pertain to younger adults who have disabilities and are perceived in a similarly dependent position as those 65 or older.

Assessing Cases of Elder Abuse and Neglect

Although a number of qualitative and quantitative instruments are available for assessing elder abuse, assessment of this problem remains an extremely complicated and multifaceted process. Several factors—such as ageism, disease in old age, the impact of multiple factors on health professionals' decision-making processes, and the autonomy of the elderly person—greatly affect assessment outcome (Fulmer, 1989).

Refer to the cases below. These four scenarios provide examples of possible mistreatment.* Try to determine the level of abuse and neglect and devise a plan of action for each situation.

Consider the following questions in each case:

1. How would you evaluate the following situations and relationships: good, tolerable, bad, neglectful, abusive (or any combination of these)?
2. How would you suggest handling each of these situations?
3. What would you want to know before making a decision?
4. Where would you go for further information about each situation and relationship (e.g., other members of health care team, other family members, neighbors and/or significant others, resource persons within community)?

Case Study 1: *The Cairns Family*

Mrs. Cairns is caring for her 78-year-old mother-in-law (Mrs. Cairns, senior) at home. Mrs. Cairns describes situations in which Mrs. Cairns senior makes nasty remarks, throws water in her face, and "purposely" smears feces all over the bathroom wall. She describes a frustrating moment when she called her husband at work and said, "If you don't come home immediately and take care of your mother, I'm going to set her in the middle of Mainstreet Blvd." Mrs. Cairns has reached a saturation point in caring for her mother-in-law. She describes kicking a box around the backyard whenever her frustration level peaks. She wants to place her mother-in-law in a nursing home but the family cannot afford to do so.

Evaluation: Bad situation, potentially abusive relationship
Things to know: What is Mr. Cairn's perception of situation? What resources are available? Is respite care possible?

---

* These cases were adapted from ones originally developed by Veronica Rempusti, MS, PhD.

Case Study 2: *Mr. Benjamin*

The home-care nurse visits 85-year-old Mr. Benjamin in his room, located in a small shacklike building behind his son's home. Dishes half-filled with food are scattered throughout the room. There are no plumbing facilities, nor are beverages available to Mr. Benjamin. The nurse was called to see Mr. Benjamin because his Foley catheter is not draining. As the RN inserts a new Foley catheter into Mr. Benjamin, a roach crawls up her leg. Mr. Benjamin refuses to be taken out of "his room" and placed in a nursing home, fearing he will never see his son again.

Evaluation: Bad situation, neglectful relationship
Things to know: Who are Mr. Benjamin's caregivers? What are their perceptions? What alternatives and interventions are available to the nurse?
Thing to do: Report to the board of health

Case Study 3: *The Stone Family*

Mrs. Stone is caring for her husband who is partially paralyzed post cardiovascular accident. She has related a history of being physically and psychologically abused by her husband throughout their 40 years of marriage, and even now he attempts to grab and slap her. She describes an incident that occurred when her husband was attempting to walk down their hallway at home, holding on to the wall. She laughed as she told this story and stated, "I just stuck out my foot and tripped him and watched him fall." Mrs. Stone is the only caregiver available to care for her husband. He is a veteran.

Evaluation: Overt abuse/40-year abusive relationship
Things to consider: Placement at VA nursing home/respite care; counseling for Mrs. Stone

Case Study 4: *The Stanskis Family*

The Stanskises live in a trailer they have owned for the last 20 years; they have been married for 60 years and have no children nor immediate family in this part of the country. Mr. Stanskis is obese, partially paralyzed, and moves about the trailer in a wheelchair. Mrs. Stanskis is extremely thin and frail with a history of anemia and vertigo. The centerpiece on their kitchen table is a serving platter filled with medication containers. Mrs. Stanskis assists Mr. Stanskis in and out of bed and with his ADLs. A nurse was called to see this couple because Mrs. Stanskis was reported to have multiple bruises on her body, and it was suspected that Mr. Stanskis had abused her.

Evaluation: Poor/bad situation, good relationship
Things to consider: Homemaker services; meals-on-wheels; supervised recreation therapy to get them outside cramped quarters.

It takes both information and sensitivity to assess a caregiving situation and evaluate it on a continuum from good to abusive. Obtain diagnostic information, uncover legal and ethical issues, and consider family cultural values and expectations. Information is not always clearcut, judgments are somewhat subjective, impressions and decisions are subject to change as information changes. Consider your own values—to what extent will they (should they) influence decisions? How do health care providers deal with situations that conflict with their own values, but avoid getting stuck in the decision-making process? For example, health professionals and caregivers often get bogged down weighing their values and diagnostic information evenly and vacillating between two perspectives. Finally, remember the importance of having information about the caregiver's roles, responsibilities, and stresses in addition to understanding the elder's needs in order to make constructive suggestions that have a good possibility of being implemented.

Caregiving can be rewarding and, at the same time, stressful. Very often the primary caregivers suffer from the burden of responsibility they have assumed but, for a variety of reasons, ignore the effects of this suffering on their own health and well-being. Caregiver stress can have serious consequences both for the caregivers, whose health may be endangered by neglect and exhaustion, and for the frail elders, who may become victims of abuse and neglect.

When frail elders are part of an informal caregiving system—especially when they depend on one family member (typically a spouse, daughter, daughter-in-law, or son) for activities of daily living—the system itself must be strong and healthy if quality care is to be delivered and maintained. If the system is impaired, intervention from health care providers may be appropriate.

Some ways Health-care providers can intervene to reduce stress and improve the functioning of the caregiving system include:

- arranging for formal services to provide respite care
- instructing caregivers about the importance of not neglecting their own health
- suggesting that caregivers learn about time management techniques, such as budgeting time, delegating responsibility to others, and setting limits
- encouraging and facilitating family conferences and open discussion of everyone's needs, responsibilities, and capabilities before making decisions
- putting caregivers in touch with support groups

Working effectively with other members of the interdisciplinary team in making assessments and decisions is important. Fulmer (1989) suggests that the most successful approach to assessment of suspected abuse is the multidisciplinary team process because it facilitates the efficient analysis of several different layers of patient information (e.g., medical record review, patient and family assessments, physical examination) by providing the necessary expertise.

Developing Action Plans to Improve Discharge Planning: Part II

Complete Part II of your action plans for improving discharge planning at your institution. In Part II of the action plan, identify outcome objectives and strategies related to your vision statement. An outcome *objective* is a statement of (a) the desired impact of the project on institutional practices and policies related to discharge planning, (b) patient outcomes after discharge, or (c) health care provider knowledge, attitudes, and practices related to discharge planning and/or gerontology. A sample objective might be "to reduce by 10% the number of elderly patients readmitted to this hospital within 6 months of discharge." A *strategy* is a general method or overall approach for meeting one's outcome objectives. Strategies for meeting the objective above might include implementing a discharge planning protocol for elderly patients and documenting the number of patients receiving that protocol and the number who are readmitted within 6 months of discharge. A copy of the action plan worksheet is included at the end of this chapter.

SUMMARY

The Key points in this chapter are:

1.   In assessing the continuing-care needs of the elderly, it is critical to look at the caregiving system, and particularly at what family members are doing or would be able and willing to do to provide assistance.

2.   For impaired elders who are receiving long-term care from an informal caregiver, it is critical to understand the caregiver's needs and capabilities as well as those of the elder person.

3.   Nurses can help impaired elders and informal caregivers develop or revise a caregiving system by exploring options for providing care that respond to the needs, abilities, and resources of both parties and recommending utilization of those community resources that the discharge planning team has determined to be good, affordable, and available to supplement informal caregiving.

4.   As a member of the multidisciplinary discharge team, the nurse plays an essential role in assessing suspected cases of elder abuse.

CLINICAL EXERCISE

Select a patient and conduct a caregiver assessment in preparation for discharge. As part of the assessment

1.   Describe the elder–family caregiver dyad: Which member is the primary caregiver? What are the essentials of the family dynamics? What resources and supports does the family have?
2.   Describe the situation requiring intervention.
3.   Develop a plan for intervention.
4.   Describe how they implemented the plan and the outcome.

REFERENCES

Brody, E. M. (1985). Parent care as a normative family stress. *The Gerontologist, 25,* 19–29.

Colerick, E. J., & George, L. K. (1986). Predictors of institutionalization among caregivers of patients with Alzheimer's disease. *Journal of the American Geriatrics Society, 34,* 1986, 493–498.

Commonwealth of Massachusetts. (1995). *Massachusetts General Laws Annotated Part I.* Administration of the government Title II. Executive and Administrative Officers of the Commonwealth. Chapter 19A, p. 1. Department of Elder Affairs. St. Paul: West Publishing.

Fulmer, T. T. (1989). Mistreatment of elders: Assessment, diagnosis, and intervention. *Nursing Clinics of North America, 24,* 707–716.

Goldstein, V., Regnery, G., & Wellin, E. (1981, January). Caretaker role fatigue. *Nursing Outlook,* pp. 24–30.

Kleeman, K. M. (1988). Family systems adaption. In F. D. Cardona, P. D. Hurn, R. J. Bastnagel-Mason, A. M. Scanlon-Schipp, & S. W. VerseBerry (Eds.), *Trauma nursing from resuscitation through rehabilitation.* Philadelphia: Saunders.

Mezey, M. D., Rauckhorst, L. H., & Stokes, S. A. (1993). *Health assessment of the older individual.* New York: Springer Publishing Co.

Noelker, L. S., & Poulshock, S. W. (1982). *The effects on families of caring for impaired elderly in residence.* Cleveland, OH: The Benjamin Rose Institute.

Silverstone, B., & Hyman, H. K. (1976). *You and your aging parent.* New York: Pantheon.

Staab, A. S., & Lyler, M. A. (1990). *Manual of geriatric nursing.* Glenview, IL: Scott Foresman.

United States House of Representatives, Subcommittee on Human Services of the Select Committee on Aging. (1987). *Exploding the myths: Caregiving in America.* Washington, DC: U. S. Government Printing Office.

Winger, J. M., Hubbard, R., & Campbell, J. (1992). Family responses to critical care. In T. T. Fulmer & M. K. Walker (Eds.), *Critical care nursing of the elderly* (pp. 306–330). New York: Springer Publishing Co.

SUGGESTED READINGS

Quayhagen, M., & Quayhagen, M. (1988). Alzheimer's stress: Coping with the caregiving role, *The Gerontologist, 28,* 391–396.

Rempusheski, V. F., & Phillips, L. R. (1988, January–February). Elders versus caregivers: Games they play. *Geriatric Nursing,* pp. 30–34.

ACTION PLAN WORKSHEET PART II: OBJECTIVES AND STRATEGIES

Outcome objectives and strategies related to my vision statement:

Outcome Objectives	Related Strategies

* *Note*: The Action Plan Worksheet was adapted from one originally developed by Christine Blaber, MEd; and Kimberly Dash, MPH, Education Development Center, Inc., under a grant from the U.S. Department of Education.

Chapter 5

ASSESSMENT OF THE POSTDISCHARGE ENVIRONMENT

LEARNING OBJECTIVES

At the end of the chapter, readers will be able to:

1. Determine how the community provides for the basic needs of its elderly citizens, including requirements for food, shelter, and social support
2. Describe how the community can meet the needs of the frail elderly
3. Conduct a home and nursing home assessment
4. Evaluate characteristics of service provision in the community, home, and nursing home, determining which functional supports are provided for the elderly and which are not
5. Begin to categorize different environments for geriatric care according to their ability to facilitate or limit patient performance and to match patients with appropriate settings
6. Link with discharge planners, social workers, and others involved in the continuing-care process in the home institution and in the community

Most health professionals are committed to helping the elderly remain in their communities as long as possible. Yet, as the number of frail elderly discharged from the hospital increases, the demand on community support services will also increase. As Waters (1987) has found, the level of dependency for most elderly is even greater at the time of discharge than immediately prior to their hospital admission. Thus, it is important that these elderly be referred to appropriate community services and to their family physicians prior to discharge, so that community and home supports can be in place on the day of discharge from the hospital (Jackson, 1990).

A comprehensive assessment of the home, community, and nursing home options prior to discharge can help nurses avoid a hasty choice made during hospital discharge. In assessing the home, community, or nursing home environment, nurses should be aware that the elderly are more vulnerable to the environment than the young. They should also be aware of the ways in which the patients' physical and mental status interact with their environment. Even if nurses cannot visit the patient's home or community it is important that they understand how this information provides a more complete picture of the patient's well-being and continuing care needs. With that broader understanding of patient needs, nurses are able to work more effectively with the interdisciplinary discharge planning team to match patients with appropriate services after discharge.

Criteria that may be used in assessing the community and home setting include provisions for (a) physical needs for adequate food, clothing, and shelter; (b) physical and psychological safety; (c) positive quality of life; and (d) continued social participation by older adults who wish to remain within the mainstream of social life (Mezey, Rauckhorst, & Stokes, 1993).

The chapter opens with a discussion of community assessment. With a strong emphasis on services, criteria to be included in assessing the community and ways that community characteristics affect the well-being of elderly patients after discharge from the hospital are considered. The section on community assessment is followed by one on home assessment and determining how well the patient will be able to manage at home after hospital discharge. A case study is presented for readers to practice making recommendations for discharge, focusing on home assessment and finding appropriate community services for the patient in the case study. The case study is followed by a review of nursing home assessment that describes some of the practical and emotional considerations and the specific steps involved in selecting a nursing home. A second case study presents the possibility of discharge to a nursing home.

THE COMMUNITY ASSESSMENT

Making a community assessment is, in some ways, similar to making a nursing diagnosis. The nurse reviews pertinent information about the community and neighborhood in which the patient lives and determines from that information how the patient's environment will either inhibit or facilitate the patient's performance in relation to basic and instrumental activities of daily living and social interaction. Based on the environmental information, the nurse and other members of the discharge planning team then try to match the patient with the least restrictive environment, or the one that will allow for optimum patient performance free from environmental hazards and risks.

Characteristics one might consider in a community assessment are specified in the following list (adapted from Mezey, Rauckhorst, & Stokes, 1993):

Overall Features
Climate

Topography

Open space or green space

Roadways

Noise

Urban, rural, or suburban

Economic base

Population Characteristics
Proportion of elderly

Socioeconomic status or characteristics of the population

Diversity: age, sex, ethnic distribution

Environmental and Safety Conditions
Crosswalks

Lighting

Traffic lights

Service Facilities
Public library

Banks

Post office

Food stores

Pharmacy

Clothing stores

Health clinics

Physicians

Visiting nurses

Home-care services

Ambulance

Social security office

Senior centers

Outreach services

Movie theaters

Parks

Places of worship

Transportation (cars, taxis, subway, or bus)

Environmental and Safety Conditions

Traffic flow

Police

Fire

Crime rate

Pollution

Service Facilities

Area Agencies on Aging

State offices of elder affairs

Public health departments

Housing agencies

Legal and financial services

Mental health programs

HMOs

Adult day-care programs

DISCUSSION QUESTIONS

Although formal resources can and do provide many essential services to the elderly, the primary source of help to most impaired elders is the people who are close to them: the relatives, friends, and neighbors who are in touch with them and may provide a great deal of their care. Recognizing and supporting caring relationships should be incorporated into any discharge plan.

General knowledge about a community can often be obtained from the patient or other local contacts. In any case, consider what the presence or absence of the environmental characteristics listed above imply about a particular community. For example: A community with a poor economic base is likely to have fewer services for the elderly. A community with a thriving industrial or commercial base may contribute to a high quality of life for the elderly because of the availability of a variety of services to choose from; however, more industry could also mean more pollution and more traffic for the elderly who live near the manufacturing facilities.

Ask yourself how the presence or absence of these environmental characteristics would affect the well-being of the elderly patient after discharge from the hospital. The presence of heavy traffic along wide boulevards, for example, is hazardous to those elderly who need to get around on foot and move slowly across the street. Scarcity of home-care services in some communities prevent the elderly from getting the care they need after discharge. For elderly with minimal mobility and transportation, services for food and clothing should ideally be located close by. A greater concentration of elderly may encourage proliferation of services for elderly in that neighborhood.

The elderly are generally more vulnerable to the environment than the young. The degree to which their level of function is impaired also determines how the environment will affect them. Discharge planners and members of the hospital social service department are likely to play a major role in community, home, and nursing home assessment and also in matching patients with appropriate services in the community.

THE HOME ASSESSMENT

Home assessment enables the nurse to determine how well the patient is managing at home. It involves assessing both the psychosocial and physical properties of the home environment. It helps the nurse identify any apparent needs that were not identified within the hospital and match resources to meet those needs. It also identifies whether the resources in place are meeting the needs of the elderly patient and whether informal supports are working. This section will review and discuss the criteria used in conducting a home assessment. Home-care options will be presented in greater detail in Chapter 6.

The most critical components of the home assessment are the physical and psychosocial environments. Safety of the physical environment is particularly important, since injuries constitute the sixth leading cause of death in people over age 75 (Kay & Tideiksaar, 1990). Most of these injuries are caused by accidents in the home. Falls are responsible for a disproportionate amount of injury, and elders are at risk to fall and injure themselves because of age-related changes and diseases that impair functioning. Yet, the physical environment can be adjusted to meet the needs of elderly patients after they are discharged from the hospital. In conducting a home assessment, the nurse or social service provider should check for the following:

Hallways, entryways, and stairs
- Flat door thresholds
- Light switches at the top and bottom of stairs
- Color contrast between the bottom and top steps of the floor
- Sufficient lighting in hallways and stairs

- Carpeting on stairs
- Easy access to the home
- Means to view and talk to a visitor without opening the door (peephole, intercom)
- Screen doors with locks
- Locks and door handles that can be easily manipulated by arthritic hands
- Deadbolt locks
- Stairs with rails
- Properly placed and working smoke detectors

Living room, dining room, and family rooms
- Secure rugs and floor coverings
- Sturdy, stationary furniture
- Accessible telephone
- Presence of non-glare light
- Adjustable lamps for sufficient lighting
- Tables 30 inches high of the ground (for patients with wheelchairs)
- Adequate heating and cooling systems

Bedrooms
- Secure rugs and floor coverings
- First floor bedroom available for someone unable to climb stairs
- Accessible telephone

Bathrooms
- Levers rather than knobs on faucets and doors (for easy manipulation)
- Presence of grabrails in the tub, toilet, or shower
- Hot water temperature set at less than 105 degrees Fahrenheit
- Non-slip material in the tub
- Shower rod that will bear weight (in case the curtain is used for support)
- Low sides on tub (to allow easy step in and step out)
- Medications labeled in clear print
- Unexposed pipes or radiators

Kitchen and laundry areas
- Stove controls in the front (to avoid reaching over the burners)
- Adequate ventilation
- Adequate storage
- Surfaces at appropriate height
- Accessible laundry
- Safe and unexposed electrical wiring

Outdoors
- Well-lighted entry
- Good drainage
- Symbolic barriers to the home, such as shrubs and fences
- Locks and break-resistant glass on ground-level windows
- Clear and smooth walkway to the home

The psychosocial environment can increase feelings of independence, self-worth, safety, and control, and improve mental functioning, social interaction, and communication. In conducting a home assessment the nurse or social service provider should check for the following:

- List of emergency phone numbers
- Ambient temperature
- Worksaving devices (e.g., dishwashers)
- Familiar and secure surroundings
- House in a secure neighborhood
- Neighbors look out for one another
- Stimulating home environment (pets, decor, family, neighbors, visitors)
- Healthy roles and relationships
- Adequate non-glare light throughout the house
- Amplification devices on phones
- Adequate privacy for the elder patient
- Adequate privacy for caregiver

Refer to the case study below.* Try to find the right community resources for an individual patient. Make recommendations for Mr.

---

* This case was adapted from one originally developed by Jane Matlaw, LKSW, ACSW, and Bonnie Jean Teitleman, MSW.

Katz's discharge plan, focusing specifically on his psychosocial home environment and finding appropriate community services for him.

Case Study: *Mr. Katz*

Mr. Katz, age 72, was admitted to a nearby neurology service with exacerbation of his Parkinson's disease. At the time of admission, he was confined to a wheelchair. His speech was garbled, his hands shook so much that he could not feed himself and he needed considerable help with daily activities. He was significantly depressed as well, with anhedonia, early morning awakenings, ruminations, hopelessness and suicidal ideation. There was a question of dementia.

The social worker learned that Mr. Katz is a Jewish man, who came to this country with his wife of 45 years and only daughter 20 years ago to escape the anti-Semitism in his country of origin. At the time of their emigration, Mr. Katz was a successful engineer, but the family had to leave behind most of their money and belongings. A few years after their arrival in the United States, the daughter, Susan, went to college, where she met and married a wealthy man. Mr. Katz and his wife live with their daughter and son-in-law in their guest house.

Mr. Katz developed Parkinson's disease within two years of his arrival to the United States. Described by his family as a proud, haughty, and independent man, he became depressed upon learning the diagnosis and prognosis of his illness. Further, he was unable to find employment in this country that was commensurate with the profession he had left behind. The English language was difficult for him. And although he eventually found work, the family suffered a loss of status, money, and profession.

Moreover, Mr. and Mrs. Katz had a stormy marital relationship. When Mr. Katz was well, Mrs. Katz became overly dependent and demanded and received much attention from her husband and daughter. She was a self-described incest survivor who had seen a psychiatrist intermittently for years. Mr. Katz had once used work as an escape from his wife's demands, but as he became less functional, he spent more time at home. This resulted in marital conflict. Mrs. Katz resented their role reversal, having to take care of her husband, while Mr. Katz was humiliated by his need for assistance with personal care. His wife hovered, treating Mr. Katz like a child. Inarticulate because of the paralysis, he hit her and she called the police. Such outbursts and resulting police intervention embarrassed the daughter and son-in-law.

During Mr. Katz's hospital course, his medications were adjusted. He received consultations from occupational therapy, physical therapy, psychiatry, nutrition, GI, neurology and social work. Because of the language difficulties, the recent move to a separate apartment, and poor communication, Mr. Katz had become quite isolated. As the work-up progressed, it became obvious that Mrs. Katz's inability to tolerate the burden of his care was the real reason for his hospital admission. One particularly odious task for Mrs. Katz involved Mr. Katz's bowel regimen. Apparently he alternated between constipation and diarrhea, depending on his diet and use of unrecommended over-the-counter medications. He was often unable to get to the bathroom in time.

At the end of the work-up, Mr. Katz was functionally the same. The nurse and the social worker called a family meeting to plan continuing care after discharge.

Questions to Consider

1. Why do you think Mr. Katz was depressed?

2. What would you recommend for his depression?

3. How would you assess the marital relationship? How do you think it affected Mr. Katz?

4. What options might you consider to address the problems in the family (marital relationship, relationship with daughter and her family)?

5. How would you assess a question of abuse, for either wife or husband?

6. What community services would be most appropriate for Mr. Katz?

7. What would you recommend to this family?

THE NURSING HOME ASSESSMENT

Practical and Emotional Considerations

Considering a nursing home is one of the most emotionally difficult decisions elderly people and their families ever face. Family members may feel they are abandoning their relatives and putting their lives in the hands of strangers who could be indifferent, cold, and hostile. The truth is that many good nursing homes do exist throughout the country, utilized by families who love their relatives very much but who, for a variety of reasons, have concluded that the elderly relative's needs can be better met in a nursing home than in any other setting.

The following indications suggest that it may be appropriate for a patient to at least consider moving to a nursing home:

1. There are times when it is extremely difficult for informal caregivers to manage or arrange care for the patient.
2. The current caregivers have difficulty attending to the patient's basic daily needs.
3. It is difficult to find and pay people to provide home care for the patient.
4. The patient's medical condition includes at least two of the following: dementia, incontinence, and a broken hip.
5. The patient's primary physician thinks a nursing home is advisable. (Be aware, however, that some physicians are not familiar with all alternatives to nursing homes such as home-care services.)
6. The caregiver's health is being impaired or environmental stresses increase.

Selecting a Nursing Home

The ultimate decision regarding nursing home care rests with the patient; and when the patient is judged not competent to make that decision, the family or appointed guardian will make it. Nurses can play a key role by helping older individuals and their families explore options ahead of time. There are four easy steps to follow in selecting a nursing home (Mezey et al., 1993):

1. Identify financial resources and barriers
2. Identify the kinds of care available
3. Identify and narrow down options
4. Compare available facilities to find the best match

Patients' financial resources essentially determine their options. If patients are able to afford private nursing home care, they have several care options. However, many patients cannot afford private nursing home care and must rely on nursing homes that are approved for reimbursement under Medicare. Medicare coverage is limited to posthospital care up to 100 days in an approved nursing facility for conditions that require skilled nursing services. The nurse or social worker should refer patients with limited resources to their local Social Security office, Department of Social Services office (for welfare), Area Agency on Aging, and/or the Medicaid office for assistance in applying for Medicaid (Mezey et al., 1993).

Three levels of nursing home care are widely available, sometimes within the same facility. *Custodial care* is available for people who don't require nursing care but who need assistance with such things as hygiene and meals. *Intermediate care* exists for people who do not need 24-hour nursing care but can no longer live alone. *Skilled nursing* is for people who need intensive round-the-clock monitoring and whose nursing care is directed by a doctor. When recommending nursing homes it is important to know what kinds of care are provided and to keep in mind that the patient's long-term needs are often custodial rather than medical.

Patients and families should identify and narrow down the options by familiarizing themselves with the nursing homes in their area. They may want to speak with physicians, social workers, friends, or family who know more about specific nursing homes. Since many patients depend on Medicare, they may also want to determine whether the nursing homes are approved for reimbursement under Medicare or Medicaid. Once patients become nursing home residents, they may eventually become eligible for Medicaid as well, if they are not eligible already.

Prospective patients and/or families should compare available facilities along with asking questions about the following parameters (Mezey et al., 1993, p. 201):

- Admission standards
- Discharge policies
- Monetary arrangements
- Room assignments and changes
- Policies regarding holding rooms if residents are hospitalized or take a vacation
- Policies concerning the amount and type of personal possessions that can be brought in
- Care of valuables and precautions against theft
- Policies and procedures to protect the privacy of residents
- Visiting hours and administrative flexibility in unusual circumstances
- Policies and schedule regarding bedtime, mealtime, and frequency of bathing
- Procedures for dealing with emergencies and life-threatening illness
- Policies regarding pets

Case Study: *Mrs. Sullivan*

Mrs. Sullivan was a 91-year-old widow and a retired real estate broker. She was admitted to the hospital from her home with a mild cerebrovascular accident. Prior to admission, Mrs. Sullivan lived at home and was in touch with the local senior home-care provider, which sent a homemaker to her house once per week. A nurse from the Visiting Nurse Association (VNA) had been seeing her monthly for her hypertension, and a social worker had been unsuccessfully attempting to have Mrs. Sullivan disclose her finances because she had refused to pay for any services. Mrs. Sullivan was a spirited woman who looked considerably younger than her age. She suffered from selective deafness and occasional incontinence.

Shortly after her admission, the social worker was contacted by a neighbor who called to describe Mrs. Sullivan's home and plead for her to be assisted in finding a nursing home. The neighbor reported that the apartment was filthy, with "garbage piled to the ceilings." Apparently Mrs. Sullivan refused to allow the homemaker to remove it.

Over the years, Mrs. Sullivan had relied increasingly on her neighbors. She called them and demanded grocery delivery. She often refused to pay, which angered some enough to stop helping. Others, however, felt she would suffer without this help, so they continued to provide food. Mrs. Sullivan had only ill words for these people, believing they were trying to steal her money.

Mrs. Sullivan's family was small and not close knit. Her sister lived in the same building, but they had not spoken in years. She had one son, who lived in another state and visited infrequently. The VNA social worker reported a number of attempts to communicate with the son; he failed to respond or write back.

As Mrs. Sullivan grew stronger and the social worker gathered this information about family and functioning, the need for a nursing home seemed clear. Mrs. Sullivan could occasionally get out of bed to the commode, but just as often did not. The nursing staff became angry with her because she demanded service for things she could do for herself. She continued to refuse nursing home placement.

The social worker thought Mrs. Sullivan was a level III candidate (i.e., required assistance or supervision from another person and equipment or device) since she could be more independent in her ADL and could walk with a walker. Her mental status was superficially quite good, although she was clearly rigid in her thinking and had poor long- and short-term memory and judgment. She did not appear to appreciate the staff's concerns for her well-being. An evaluation by occupational therapy found her safety awareness to be extremely limited. She forgot that she left a stove on, and she could not see well enough to guard against falls. In fact, she had several falls in the hospital, which she quickly forgot.

Mrs. Sullivan's care providers from the community came in to try and persuade her to accept placement in a nursing home. They were unsuccessful. Her doctors, nurses, and physical and occupational therapists met almost daily with her—again without success. Finally, a psychiatric evaluation was requested. If Mrs. Sullivan was found to be significantly compromised, a court could find her incompetent and begin proceedings to obtain a guardian. The psychiatrist, however, found her to be functioning sufficiently and able to make decisions, even if they were poor ones.

Mrs. Sullivan's sister called daily for an update and expressed the hope that Mrs. Sullivan would "be put away for good." She declined to assume any responsibility, saying it was the son's job. Mrs. Sullivan, who was clearly comfortable in the hospital milieu, procrastinated by saying, "Tomorrow I'll think about a nursing home, today I want to go home." She told stories of her years in real estate and how much money she had hidden away.

Now, a couple weeks after the psychiatric evaluation, the staff was still frustrated. They did not believe Mrs. Sullivan to be safe, yet she refused placement. Previous support from the neighbors was withdrawn. In a final blow to the discharge plan, VNA refused to take Mrs. Sullivan's case again unless she had 24-hour care, which she refused to pay for.

Questions to Consider

1. What are Mrs. Sullivan's short-term care needs at discharge?

2. What options might you consider for meeting those needs?

3. What factors influence your recommendations? (For example: patient's abilities, attitudes and wishes; availability and quality of community-based resources, and patient's willingness to use them; and her own resources.)

4. What are Mrs. Sullivan's long-term care needs?

5. What options might you consider for meeting those needs?

6. What factors influence your decision?

7. What is her family's responsibility?

8. What ethical issues does this case raise? (Ethical issues in discharge planning will be covered in greater detail in Chapter 7.)

9. How might you collaborate with the social worker in this situation?

10. Once you get Mrs. Sullivan to agree to a nursing home referral, how would you proceed to find an appropriate one for her? What kinds of information would you need to collect from Mrs. Sullivan before helping her choose a nursing home?

SUMMARY

The key points of this chapter are:

1. Collaborating with the social worker or discharge planner, the nurse can play a key role by helping older individuals and their families explore community, home, and nursing home options prior to discharge.

2. In assessing the home and community environment, the nurse and other health and social service providers should be aware of how the patients' physical and mental status interacts with their environment.

3. The elderly are generally more vulnerable to the environment than the young.

CLINICAL EXERCISES

1. Investigate and document three potential community referrals for a patient in your care. Describe type and extent of service provided, patient eligibility, patient ability to pay, and appropriateness of care.

2. Select a defined community near your hospital and conduct a community diagnosis. Outline criteria for the diagnosis (or assessment) and focus on the services, in particular health and social services, available to the elderly in that community.

3. Select a long-term care facility in your community and, with one of their patients in mind, assess the care provided at that facility using the assessment form provided in Appendix A of this chapter.

REFERENCES

Jackson, M. F. (1990). Use of community support services by elderly patients discharged from general medical and geriatric medical wards. *Journal of Advanced Nursing, 15,* 157–175.

Kay, A. D., & Tideiksaar, L. (1990). Falls and gait disorders. In W. B. Abrams, & R. Berkow (Eds.), *The Merck manual of geriatrics* (p. 52). Rahway, NJ: Merck, Sharp & Dohme.

Mezey, M. D., Rauckhorst, L. H., & Stokes, S. A. (1993). *Health assessment of the older individual.* New York: Springer Publishing Co.

Waters, K. R. (1987). Outcomes of discharge from hospital for elderly people. *Journal of Advanced Nursing, 12,* 347–355.

SUGGESTED READING

Blazyk, S., & Canaban, M. M. (1985, November–December). Therapeutic aspects of discharge planning. *Social Work,* pp. 489–496.

APPENDIX A

Long-Term Care Facility Assessment Form

Name _____   Date Visited _____

Address _____   Phone Number _____

Level   I   II   III   IV   Chronic Rehab   No. of beds _____

Room Rates _____   Owner _____

Public Transportation _____

_____

Administrator _____   Director of Nursing _____

Contact Person _____   Application necessary?   Yes _____   No _____

Percentage of patients accepted on Medicaid _____%   Will accept your patients? Yes _____   No _____

Please check if the following are offered:

Ostomy care	_____	Psychiatry	_____	Social worker:	_____
Bowel/blad prog	_____	Dental	_____	MSW: Consult _____ Staff _____	
Tube feedings:	_____	Calendar of activs	_____	Counseling	_____
NG _____ G _____ J	_____	Community vols	_____	Screening	_____
IVs	_____	Transportation	_____	Family work	_____
Indwelling caths	_____	Resident council	_____	Medicaid eligibility	_____
Hyperalimentation	_____	Speech therapy	_____	Groups:	_____
Ventilators	_____	PT _____ OT	_____	Describe:	_____

Facility accepts: Wanderers _____   Psych. patients _____   Past ETOH history _____

Management Problems _____   Dialysis   Patients _____

Comments:_____

_____

_____

Nursing inservice/staff edu _____

Nursing coverage (agency?) _____

Medical Director _____ Hospital Backup _____

Are patients able to retain their own physician?   Yes _____   No _____

Physical description of facility _____

Types of rooms: Private _____   2 Bed _____   3 Bed _____   4 Bed _____

Elevators: Yes _____   No _____

Does facility smell of urine?   Yes _____   No _____

Comments

Appearance of patients

Facility's strengths

Facility's limitations

_____

_____

Evaluators

Source: Developed by Jane Matlaw and Nancy Zarle, Beth Israel Hospital, Boston, MA

Chapter **6**

MATCHING PATIENTS WITH AVAILABLE RESOURCES

LEARNING OBJECTIVES

At the end of this chapter, readers will be able to:

1. Describe the various sources of support for the elderly patient at discharge
2. Explain patient eligibility requirements for different services and complete appropriate admissions procedures and requirements
3. Identify funding sources for services to the discharged patient and understand procedures for reimbursement
4. Identify and overcome individual and system challenges to creating high-quality discharge plans

The purpose of this chapter is to pull together informal and formal supports available to the elderly and outline the procedures for matching the needs of the elder with these available services. The chapter addresses the forces that impinge on that process, namely, the impact of Medicare's Prospective Payment System on health care patients, providers, and institutions. It also delineates steps to follow in planning for discharge when an elderly patient will require skilled medical care in the home environment.

First, there is review of support systems available to elderly patients at the time of hospital discharge, including family and community support systems. The role finances play in discharge planning is explained. Patient funding sources, whether from family, Medicare, Medicaid, or other insurers, are identified as the essential determinant of what type of care may be available and affordable to the frail elderly after hospital discharge.

Home-care resources are examined next, especially the increasing availability of skilled medical services to the elderly in their homes. Other areas covered include finding home health care agencies and planning home care. Topics include determining the range of services needed, matching resources with needs, and providing an optimal environment.

Case studies are presented, for practice. Questions will guide readers in developing a discharge plan, describing system challenges and ways of overcoming them, identifying resources, and identifying least restrictive environments for each case.

Discharge planning for the elderly begins at hospital admission with a complete physical and functional assessment of the elderly patient. The period of hospitalization itself should be viewed as a discrete event in the ongoing process of planning continuing care. During the patient's stay it is essential to think about how to meet the patient's needs outside the hospital. As part of this process, nurses should conduct or arrange for a community and home assessment prior to discharge (see chapter 5). In addition, nurses should maintain or develop a comprehensive list of community resources available for meeting not only the patient's basic needs but also those needs that require skilled medical assistance. An understanding of constraints and access for matching needs with resources will help ensure a successful plan.

SOURCES OF SUPPORT FOR THE ELDERLY

The Family

Families are the primary source of support for the elderly during the posthospitalization period (Jones, Densen, & Brown, 1989). Women are usually the primary caregivers for the frail elderly. When the husband is functionally disabled, the wife usually becomes the primary caregiver, if she is able. Daughters and daughters-in-law who live nearby also assist with care on a day-to-day basis, while sons may provide services such as financial help and transportation.

The long-term health care needs of the elderly are primarily custodial. Custodial care is unskilled care. It may include help in walking, getting in and out of bed, eating, dressing, and housekeeping. Unfortunately, this kind of care is not covered by Medicare.

In many cases, the family also assumes responsibility for providing direct care for the older person. Because skilled medical services are not always available or accessible, the family must perform the kinds of services offered by these agencies.

However, the family is not always able to take care of the elderly patient or provide the kind of quality care needed. The number of elderly who need formal and skilled home health care is increasing, due to the rising numbers of very old persons, the changing availability of family supports, and the impact of policies such as the Prospective Payment System (Gornick & Hall, 1988). When the elderly need skilled care or formal assistance, they often turn to home health care services.

When family members are not available, the elderly must seek assistance from the community or from alternative care facilities. The primary source of formal services for older persons during the posthospitalization period is Medicare home health care. As average lengths of hospital stays among the elderly have decreased, the use of Medicare home health care has increased significantly (National Center for Health Statistics, 1988).

The Community

The broader political, legal, and economic climate can affect discharge planning and continuing care for elderly patients. Since 1932 major legislation, influenced by economic and demographic changes, has produced a broad array of home health and supportive services available to the elderly patient in need of long-term care. Legislation relevant to discharge planning and continuing care of the elderly is described below.

1. The Social Security Act (1932) increased financial security for the elderly.

2. The amendments to the Social Security Act (1950s) allowed vendor payments to nursing homes caring for the elderly.

3. The First White House Conference on Aging (1951) brought

visibility to problems of the aged and launched national level policy making to address problems of the aged. (White House Conferences on Aging have been held each decade since that time.)

4.   Medicare (1965), title 18 of the Social Security Act, established medical insurance for all older adults; and the federal government began to set standards for institutions providing care for the aged.

5.   Medicaid (1965), title 19 of the Social Security Act, made available acute illness care to people unable to afford it and increased federal regulation of hospitals and nursing homes. Proliferation of nursing homes is associated with this legislation.

6.   Title 20 of the Social Security Act (1965) made available in-home services for medically indigent elderly through social service agencies.

7.   The Older Americans Act (1965) established aging networks throughout the states, introduced the concept of a "focal point" for services to the aged, and funded noninstitutional health services external to the social services agencies.

Health-supportive services, such as meal preparation, shopping, light and heavy housecleaning, health management, personal care, transportation and escorting are funded under title 20 of the Social Security Act and the Older American Act.

8.   Medicare reform legislation and changes in regulations (1972) established intermediate care facilities as a new type of reimbursed nursing-home care.

9.   The Omnibus Reconciliation Act (1981) established Medicare reform, waiving 3-day prior hospitalization requirements for extended care benefits and removing the limit on number of home health visits allowed.

10.   The Tax Equity and Fiscal Responsibility Act (TEFRA, 1982) introduced prospective reimbursement for hospitals under Medicare and also initiated promulgation of regulations for hospice to allow reimbursement for hospice care under Medicare and Medicaid.

11.   The Medicare Catastrophic Coverage Act (1988) expanded coverage to protect the elderly from catastrophic costs associated with acute illness and provided insurance coverage for prescription drugs. Unfortunately it forced many elderly to pay higher premiums associated with Medicare Part B.

Thus, there are various funding sources for the many home health and supportive services available to elderly patients. Note that skilled services such as medical services, home nursing services, personal care, and day hospital services are funded by Medicaid (title 19 of the Social Security Act).

The Veterans Administration and Medicare (title 20 of the *Social Security Act*) are the next major funders of skilled services. Personal-care aide services have the greatest variety of funding sources, including Medicare, Medicaid, the Social Security Act, the Administration on Aging, and the Veterans Administration.

Although each state provides social support services for the elderly, eligibility for these programs varies from state to state. Consult your state offices on aging for more information about program availability and access requirements. Local Councils on Aging and Area Agencies on Aging can also provide information about services and programs for each area of the country. It is the discharge team's responsibility to know the local eligibility requirements for community-based services (e.g., services that include meal preparation, shopping, house cleaning, health management, personal care, and transportation).

The Client

More than 70% of the retired elderly have incomes above the poverty level; however, few are "well-off." Inflation and increasing medical expenses tend to quickly deplete their incomes. In fact, 80% of an older person's income goes to basic living expenses such as food, housing, transportation, and medical care. Among the elderly, older, single women are the hardest hit because they live longer, often have been dependent non-wage earners, and have never handled financial affairs.

Two supplementary sources of income for the elderly client are social security benefits and welfare programs. Social Security benefits may be the elder's primary source of income and they include:

- Retirement checks, amount formulated from years of employment and contribution to the system
- Disability checks
- Survivor's checks

Social Security was not created to be used as income. It was originally established to act as insurance for lost potential income due to retirement. The major financial supports for old age should be derived from pension plans, investments, and private savings. However, the fact remains that for many elderly people, the only source of income is Social Security.

Welfare programs are also available to the elderly. Welfare programs were established to ensure that all Americans are able to maintain, at the minimum, a predetermined standard of living. This level is influenced by the economic conditions of the country in general. Welfare eligibility is not influenced by age, but by income and assets. The elderly, along with the visually impaired, physically challenged, and mothers with dependent children, are usually eligible. Types of welfare programs include:

- Supplemental Security Income (SSI): people 65 and older, blind or disabled with limited income are eligible
- Food Stamp program: eligibility varies from state to state
- Social Service programs: *The Older American Act* (1965) and *Medicaid title 19* pay doctor, hospital, nursing home, and other health costs of eligible poor; eligibility varies from state to state

Public benefit programs such as Medicare and Medicaid do help the elderly pay for health care; private "medigap" insurance and health maintenance organizations (HMOs) can also help the elderly afford the high cost of health care. However, even with these programs, the elderly have out-of-pocket medical expenses that can run to hundreds of dollars a year. In fact, the elderly usually pay 30% of their health care costs from their own pockets. Also, it is important to understand that the long-term care needs of most elderly people—whether they live in the community or in long-term care facilities—are primarily custodial, not medical. Except for long-term care insurance (a relatively new and expensive type of private insurance, which generally offers little help to the noninstitutionalized impaired elderly) very little assistance, from either public or private sources, is available to cover the long-term care needs of the elderly. Medicaid covers some costs for those elderly who are eligible; for the rest, the burden of paying for long-term care is borne by the elderly themselves and their families.

Medicare

Medicare Part A helps pay for "medically necessary" skilled nursing facilities or psychiatric hospital, and hospice care. Medicare Part A also pays the full cost of medically necessary home health care and 80% of approved durable medical equipment. Medically necessary home health services can include part-time visiting nurses, physical therapists, and speech therapists from a Medicare-certified agency. Medicare also covers part-time home health aide services, occupational therapy, medical services, and medical supplies. Medicare does not cover such things as private duty nursing, custodial care, full-time nursing care at home, routine tests, or drugs.

Medicare Part B helps pay for doctors' services (inpatient and outpatient services and fees), outpatient procedures, diagnostic tests, durable medical equipment such as wheelchairs, and many other services and supplies not covered under Part A. Enrollment in Part B is voluntary and carries a monthly premium.

Since January, 1993, there has been a cap on the patient's Part B cost-sharing responsibility. Physicians cannot charge more than 15% above the Medicare-approved amount for a given procedure. In addition, Medicare will cover home intravenous (IV) drug therapy with patients paying a coinsurance 20% for these IV drugs.

Supplemental Policies

Supplemental insurance policies add other health care benefits to basic (Medicare) coverage. First, medigap policies, private insurance policies designal to supplement Medicare's benefits, can fill in some of the gaps in Medicare, such as check-ups, eye exams, hearing aids, and private duty nursing. Second, health maintenance organizations (HMOs) can also fill in some of the gaps in Medicare for a fixed rate. Both insurer and health care provider, HMOs are composed of hospitals, doctors, and other health professionals who serve an enrolled group for a fixed fee, paid in advance. If an elderly patient is covered under both parts of Medicare, the HMO plan must provide or arrange for all Part A and B services. Unfortunately, most HMOs do not provide home health services. Group insurance is a third form of supplemental insurance and includes, for example, employer group insurance and association group insurance.

The Medicaid program covers doctor, hospital, nursing home, and related health costs for the eligible poor. (Eligibility requirements vary from state to state since this is a joint federal and state program.)

A variety of private health insurance policies may insure the well-to-do elderly. Some companies will reimburse the Medicare deductible. However, the monthly premium for these plans is so high that it is not worthwhile for most elderly. Long-term care insurance plans in the public and private sectors are just now emerging. As people live longer and the numbers of older people increase, insurance plans for helping them remain in their homes with skilled services will be developed.

In summary, nurses need to recognize the cost constraints of elderly persons affected by fixed incomes and lack of Medicare coverage for long-term health care services. When planning for discharge, nurses should be aware that costs can be contained by (a) enlisting services of family and friends, (b) matching patients with volunteer and community services, and (c) prescribing generic medications.

THE HOME CARE SOLUTION

The Impact of Early Discharge and the Emerging Popularity of Home Care

Due to the sharp rise in Medicare outlays—from $3 billion to $45 billion between 1967 and 1984—the Health Care Financing Administration implemented a fixed price Prospective Payment System (PPS) for inpatient services delivered to Medicare beneficiaries. The new system, based on diagnosis-related groups (DRGs), provides hospitals with a fixed reimbursement per discharge. It represents a radical shift from a multiple fee-for-service structure to a single fee-for-diagnosis structure.

What was originally intended by the federal government to reward and produce more cost-effective management of the patient, may now be producing significant changes in the health care industry. One of the more common means of reducing costs associated with patient care has been early discharge, or reduction in length of stay (Balinsky & Starkman, 1987). The introduction of the PPS and subsequent reductions in lengths of hospital stays for the elderly has affected health care's patients, providers, and institutions.

Since the advent of PPS, the number of elderly discharged from hospitals in unstable conditions has increased across the board rather than in any specific patient or hospital subgroup (Rogers et al., 1990). Because they are discharged sicker and quicker from acute-care hospitals, many elderly patients have care needs that are too complex for their families to manage and thus require formal in-home health care services.

Medicare's Prospective Payment System impacts health care providers as well. For example, physicians no longer make home visits nor do they have the time to take care of the multiple care needs of elderly patients.

The PPS has significant impact on hospitals and home care agencies. It has produced significant changes in the balance between patient care needs and service, contributing to an increase in the number of hospitals and proprietary organizations in the home care industry. Since the establishment of DRGs, there has been a 30% increase in the use of home health services (Balinsky & Starkman, 1987).

In addition, home health agencies have experienced increases in visits per patient, service provision that require multiple visits per week, and specialized services such as ventilators and home infusion therapy, which was previously not reimbursible through Medicare. Therefore, home health care agencies and their staff have had to develop new skills, especially in the area of acute care. They must accommodate more visits per patient and deal with less predictability in patient status. To cope, they develop policies that address and expand the scope of practice.

Defining Home Care

The National Association for Home Care (NAHC) defines home care as any or all of a full range of health care and social services offered to patients in their homes.

Home care is one aspect of long-term care. Long-term care services may be continuous or intermittent and are delivered to individuals who have a demonstrated need as measured by some index of functional dependency (Kane & Kane, 1981). In the past, long-term care was considered to be nursing home placement. Now, however, care in a nursing home is no longer a viable solution for many elderly. Because nursing homes are often neither accessible, available, nor desirable, many elderly are choosing to remain at home. Therefore, home care services have become part of the long-term care continuum.

There are two types of home care services. Comprehensive home health service is a plan designed by a professional nurse in cooperation with a physician. Homemaker-home health care service may be required in addition to nursing and a variety of therapies (e.g., speech, physical, occupational). It can include help with personal grooming, general housekeeping and, in some cases, escorting or accompanying clients to various health or related services.

Where to Find Home Health Care Agencies

Home health care agencies fall into the following profit-making or nonprofit categories:

- for-profit agencies that bypass licensing usually contracting with certified agencies to supply home care for them
- Nonprofit agencies run by local communities and governed by a board of directors composed of health professionals, funded by Medicare, Medicaid, private insurance companies, direct payment and/or contributions
- Hospital-based agencies that help ensure continuity of care by providing services directly when there are gaps in community services
- Community-based agencies (either nonprofit or for profit) that have increasingly entered the home care industry as a result of Medicare's PPS
- Public health and social service, whose range of services vary locally

Agency licensing for reimbursement by Medicare is carried out by individual states.

Planning Home Care

When planning home care, the important steps are to:

1. Assess health and functional status of the patient
2. Determine the range of services needed
3. Match resources with needs

4. Provide the least restrictive or optional environment
5. Support decision making
6. Help select the best long-term care arrangement
7. Assist in adjustment: guilt, relocation stress, loss of privacy and control, death

Throughout discharge planning, ask, Are data collection and patient assessments complete? Without a full knowledge base, matching will likely not be appropriate. A major goal of planning is to clearly discern all areas of maintenance and support needed to help individuals remain functional within their home environment. To do this the nurse/ discharge planner must have a complete assessment of the person's needs and know what resources are available to make appropriate referrals.

Have you identified the specific skilled nursing care needs of the patient? What are those aspects of care requiring a knowledgeable person to assist the patient with in the least restrictive environment? For examples, will the patient need dressing changes, medication (including IV) instruction, indwelling catheters, assessment, or other treatments?

Have you identified any informal supports that can meet these needs? Have you involved the patient and family in planning? Involvement of the patient and family is critical when planning what will occur in the posthospital environment. Without their active participation and agreement, there is no guarantee that the plan will be carried out. Involving the patient and family increases their understanding and should increase adherence to the plan.

By involving the patient and/or family you may also be able to identify some services they can be educated to perform themselves. For example, a number of elderly or family members can be taught to care for an indwelling Foley catheter. Involvement of family is especially important if health services will not be covered by some form of insurance and if the patient lacks the means to pay for services directly.

If patients are to remain in the home, they must be able to care for themselves when agency staff are not present. The main difference between those patients who will be able to remain in the home and those who will not is related not to health and functioning, but rather to the availability of informal supports such as family and friends. A 1979 survey conducted by the Urban Institute of various professionals frequently involved in long-term care placement decisions indicates that the absence of informal supports, rather than the unavailability of formal home-based services, was the key factor in the selection of a nursing home over other alternatives for most dependent clients and patients (Dunlop & Durman, 1979).

Have you identified which skilled support services would most likely meet an individual's needs? Matching also involves some sort of assessment of patient needs. Many states have placement requirements, and patients are matched according to degree of need. Issues of access (e.g., availability, cost, safety, and support) also need to be resolved.

Have you identified the optimal environment in which the needs can be met? Often "optimal environment" means an environment that is least restrictive. However, what is restrictive to one person may not be restrictive to another. And those environments classified as "least restrictive" are often not feasible for many elderly. In Figure 6.1, environments and corresponding services are organized by categories on a continuum of care. It is important to note that services are organized by categories for ease of presentation and that these services are not necessarily discrete. Hospice services, for example, are listed in both more restrictive and less restrictive categories. Some might also argue that housing options could be placed in the less restrictive category as well, depending on the individual establishment.

Does the patient consent to the plan? Some states now require patient signatures on the discharge plan that was developed with them. If they reject the plan then the hospital may be obliged to allow the patient to stay another day or two until it meets the patient's approval.

In sum, services to the nonhospitalized elderly should be accessible, comprehensive, and coordinated; and home-care providers and staff should be accountable and collaborative.

Refer to the cases of Mr. Martinez and Mrs. Walker to develop a discharge plan to meet the needs of these individuals.* Identify resources required and the least restrictive environment in each case.

---

* These cases were adapted from ones originally developed by Susan Burns-Tisdale, RN, MPH.

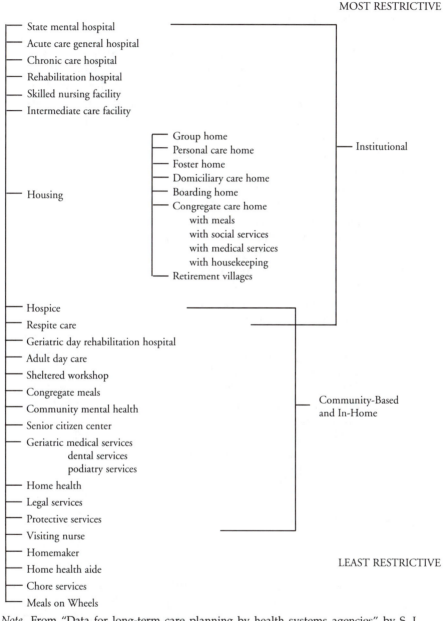

Note. From "Data for long-term care planning by health systems agencies" by S. J. Brody and C. Masciocchi, 1980, *American Journal of Public Health, 10,* ll. Copyright © The American Public Health Association. Adapted by permission.

FIGURE 6.1 Array of services.

Case Study: *Mr. Martinez*

Mr. Paul Martinez, an 85-year-old man, was rushed by ambulance to the hospital emergency department on June 10. Mr. Martinez's building superintendent telephoned the ambulance when he noticed that Mr. Martinez was having difficulty breathing. Mr. Martinez was admitted and diagnosed with exacerbation of congestive heart failure (CHF). Mr. Martinez has been in the hospital for 5 days and has responded well to treatment. He has been scheduled for discharge.

Mr. Martinez has a history of CHF and mild dementia. His clinical nurse feels that he was admitted to the hospital with exacerbated CHF because he is neither able to comply with a long list of medications nor adhere to a specialized diet. Even though she has prepared a medication chart for him to take home and has reviewed his medications with him this time, she is concerned that he will not be able to manage his medications and diet. He demonstrates noticeable difficulty remembering things. Since his wife's death in 1980, Mr. Martinez has lived alone. He has a few acquaintances in his apartment building, but is basically on his own. He says his closest companion is his dog, who's been with him since his wife's death.

Mr. Martinez is unable to leave his apartment unless assisted. He has an unsteady gait and uses a walker. He was noted to be somewhat unkempt on admission.

For food, Mr. Martinez contacts a local market which delivers to his home. He is insured through Medicare and is currently applying for Medicaid.

Questions to Consider

1. What is your discharge plan for him?

2. What individual and system challenges do you anticipate? (For example: noncompliance, medications, diet needs and restrictions, memory changes, loose social supports, impaired functional ability, saftey in apartment, and personal care needs.)

3. What would you do to overcome these challenges? (For example: follow up medication and diet needs with VNA, arrange home-

maker services for shopping and meal preparation, and assist with Medicaid application and follow up with the social services department.)

Case Study: *Mrs. Walker*

Mrs. Lillian Walker is a 68-year-old woman admitted to the hospital for failure to thrive. She was accompanied by her niece, Alice, who had been visiting her and noticed that her aunt had experienced significant weight loss and had become incontinent since her last visit 3 weeks earlier.

During her admission, Mrs. Walker was assessed by neurology and psychiatry and was diagnosed with Alzheimer's disease. She was found to be mentally competent despite obvious poor judgment.

Before her retirement 5 years ago, Mrs. Walker had worked for many years as a secretary in a law firm. She lives alone in a large home that originally belonged to her parents. She is well known in the neighborhood. In fact, neighbors contacted her niece last January to report that she was wandering about the neighborhood dressed in summer clothes.

Mrs. Walker's major source of support is her niece, Alice, who lives 2 hours away. Yet Alice has expressed concern to both the nurse and social worker about her ability to assist her aunt in meeting her aunt's needs. Alice says she has her hands full with a husband, five children, and a part-time job.

Mrs. Walker is insured by Medicare and has significant assets. She has asked to return home.

Questions to Consider

1.   What is your discharge plan for her?

2.   What individual and system challenges do you anticipate? (For example: She is unable to meet her nutritional needs and she has been reported to wander.)

3.   What would you do to overcome them? (Consider that Mrs. Walker's niece lives nearby, she has her own house, and she wants to return home.)

Developing Action Plans to Improve Discharge Planning: Part III

Complete Part III of your action plan for improving discharge planning at your institution. Part III will identify human, financial, and material resources you can call on to carry out your project. Think about resources available in the hospital and in the community. Remember that material resources such as articles on the effectiveness of certain models of discharge planning can be helpful in mustering support from hospital staff and administration. See Appendix A of chapter 6 for a suggested format for Part III of your Action Plan.

SUMMARY

The key points of this chapter are:

1.   There are a number of support systems available to elderly patients at discharge, including family, community, and patient resources.
2.   Because they are discharged early from acute care hospitals, many elders require in-home health care services. Many of these services are custodial and are therefore not covered by Medicare.
3.   Many elderly, affected by fixed incomes and lack of Medicare coverage for long-term care services, face major cost constraints upon discharge.
4.   Less restrictive environments such as the home setting, are preferable environments for discharged elders than the more restrictive institutional setting. However, those environments classified as "least restrictive" are often not feasible options for many elderly.

CLINICAL EXERCISE

Identify one challenge in the development of a patient's discharge plan and develop two strategies for responding to that challenge.

REFERENCES

Balinsky, W., & Starkman, J. L. (1987). The impact of the DRGs on the health care industry. *Health Care Management Review, 12*(3), 61–74.

Dunlop, B., & Durman, E. (1979, October). *Impact of family, professionals, and payment source on long-term care placement decisions.* Paper presented at the annual meeting of the American Public Health Association, New York City.

Gornick, M., & Hall, M. (1988). Trends in Medicare use of post-hospital care. *Health Care Financing Review, 10* (Suppl.) 27–38.

Jones, E., Densen, P., & Brown, S. (1989). Post-hospital needs of elderly people at home: Findings from an eight-month follow-up study. *Health Services Research, 24,* 643–664.

Kane, R., & Kane, R. A. (1981). *Assessing the elderly: A practical guide to measurement.* Lexington, MA: Lexington Books.

National Center for Health Statistics, Hospital Care Statistics Branch (1988). *1987 summary: National hospital discharge survey. Advance data from vital and health statistics, No. 159* (DHHS Publication No. PHS 88-1250). Hyattsville, MD: Public Health Service.

Rogers, W. H., Draper, D., Kahn, K. L., Keeler, E. B., Rubenstein, L. V., Kosecoff, J. & Brook, R. H. (1990). Quality of care before and after implementation of the DRG-based prospective payment system. *Journal of the American Medical Association, 264,* 1989–1994.

SUGGESTED READINGS

Edelstein, H., & Lang, A. (1991). Post-hospital care for older people: A collaborative solution. *The Gerontologist, 31,* 267–270.

Kass, D. I. (1987, May). Alternatives to financing home health care. *Business and Health,* pp. 16–20.

McCann, J. (1988, March). Long-term home care for the elderly: Perceptions of nurses, physicians, and primary caregivers. *Quality Review Bulletin,* pp. 66–74.

Roybal, E. R. (1987, May). Making home care a workable alternative. *Business and Health,* pp. 11–13.

APPENDIX A

Action Plan Worksheet
Part III: Human, Financial, and Material Resources

I will ask the following groups and individuals to help me implement my plan:

_____
_____
_____
_____
_____
_____
_____

Information, material, and financial resources I can call upon to implement my plan:

_____
_____
_____
_____
_____
_____
_____
_____
_____
_____
_____

* *Note*: The Action Plan Worksheet was adapted from one originally developed by Christine Blaber, MEd; and Kimberly Dash, MPH, Education Development Center, Inc., under a grant from the U.S. Department of Education.

Chapter 7

ETHICAL ISSUES IN DISCHARGE PLANNING

LEARNING OBJECTIVES

At the end of this chapter, readers should be able to:

1. Identify common ethical dilemmas in discharge planning
2. Structure and clarify ethical dilemmas associated with discharge planning
3. Strengthen their role as a patient advocate, who supports the patients' right to make as many decisions as possible for themselves

Discharge planning issues are among the major causes of moral and ethical concerns of nursing staff. Nurses are often troubled by the demoralization of older patients who fail to regain their preadmission level of functioning. Nurses are also concerned about procedures that increase patients' dependence and relegate them to nursing homes. They question whether life in an institution with a tracheotomy or gastrostomy tube is a good outcome of hospital treatment (Strumpf & Paier, 1992). Nurses ask: Is the lifesaving procedure in the best interest of the patient? It may prolong the patient's life, but the quality of that life may not meet the patient's expectations and definition of quality. Thus, a tension forms between the nurses' felt duty to do good and prevent harm to the patient and the patient's right to autonomy and self-governance. This tension of two opposing forces implies a dilemma and, as such, indicates that there will be trade-offs made in resolving that tension.

Ethical dilemmas like those mentioned above have no easy answers. Many of the earlier chapters have touched on ethical issues nurses may face when planning hospital discharge and continuing care for the frail elderly. This chapter, however, takes a closer look at identifying and dealing with dilemmas in discharge planning. It is particularly important for nurses to confront the moral and ethical dilemma of discharge planning and feel not only comfortable but skilled in raising ethical issues. Nurses must realize, however, that they are not alone in dealing with ethical problems. Under particularly troubling circumstances (such as family and staff conflict) they should seek assistance and resolution through critical discussion with the interdisciplinary discharge planning team or the hospital ethics committee, if one is available.

This chapter opens with a brief introduction to the principles and components of medical ethics. Ethics is defined as a morally acceptable process of critical thinking for making decisions. It examines the professional code of ethics, identifies ways to recognize ethical dilemmas, describes four ethical principles (autonomy, beneficence, nonmaleficence, and justice), and highlights the components of an ethical dilemma.

A comparison of two different approaches to ethical problem solving is made: the balancing approach and the philosophical approach. Readers then practice applying these two approaches by trying to solve an ethical dilemma and develop a discharge plan for a case study.

ANATOMY OF AN ETHICAL DILEMMA

To be able to resolve an ethical dilemma in discharge planning, nurses must first be able to recognize what types of situations are most likely to raise ethical concerns. The anatomy of an ethical dilemma is discussed below.

Defining Ethics

Ethics is defined as a morally acceptable process of critical thinking for making decisions. Ethics is the process by which one determines a moral solution. Ethical theory and reasoning do not solve ethical dilemmas, but provide ways of structuring and clarifying them.

Ethics in nursing is the critical examination of the moral dimension of decision making in both daily practice and policy making. At the practice level, ethical actions are based on critical thinking about one's duties and obligations as an individual nurse in relation to patients and as a member of a profession fulfilling a social contract (Aroskar, 1980). The American Nurses Association published a code of ethics for the nursing profession in 1976. Portions of the code are relevant to ethical problems encountered in discharge planning for the frail elderly. These include:

- Respecting human dignity and the uniqueness of the client without considerations of social or economic status, personal attributes, or the nature of health problems
- Protecting the patient's right to privacy while advocating for the health of both the patient and the public whenever health care and safety are affected
- Assuming responsibility and accountability for individual nursing judgments and actions
- Maintaining the integrity of the nursing profession
- Collaborating with members of the health professions and other citizens in promoting local, state, and national efforts to meet public health needs

An ethical dilemma is a conflict between moral principles. The four ethical principles considered fundamental to the relationship between health-care providers and their clients are autonomy, beneficence, nonmaleficence, and justice. Any principle can compete with any other for priority in a specific case.

Autonomy is the most frequently discussed principle in health care. It should be honored in the provision of care and can be promoted by interdisciplinary action. Autonomy is generally defined as self-governance: being one's own person without constraints by another's action or by psychological or physical limitations (Beauchamp & Childress, 1983). Kapp (1987, p. 548) defines autonomy as "the concept of self-determination and freedom, the idea that each person, to the maximum extent possible, should be permitted to make and act upon major life decisions on the basis of personal values and preferences."

The principle of autonomy grants individuals the right to consent to or refuse medical or therapeutic intervention. The act of consent should be genuinely voluntary, and there must be adequate disclosure of information. Issues of patient competence, disparities between patient acceptance and comprehension of information, and disclosure of potentially sensitive information are likely to create dilemmas of autonomy. For example, patients prone to periods of confusion are sometimes—but not always—able to understand their condition. Although competent to make decisions about their care, patients may not always comprehend the information and thus, may not always be making an informed decision. Dilemmas of disclosure, on the other hand, deal with when to provide patients with information about their conditions, even when physicians or nurses believe that the information itself might be harmful to the patient.

As Beauchamp and Childress argue, one can be autonomous and make choices autonomously without necessarily being accorded the respect due an autonomous person. Patients are often allowed to make decisions but feel as if they had been indulged in a whim. Instead, a patient's right to self-governance should be affirmed. They should be reminded that they are entitled to autonomous determination, free of imposed limitations.

The principle of autonomy does not apply to individuals unable to act in a sufficiently autonomous way because they are immature, incapacitated, ignorant, coerced, or in a position in which they can be exploited by others. Usually, the only reason to remove personal liberty is to prevent patients from harming themselves or others.

Describe conflicts you have experienced or might foresee experiencing that would involve issues of autonomy. When would autonomy *not* apply to the elderly?

Beneficence is the active promotion of good. For nurses, it is the obligation to promote a patient's health and welfare, and to help fulfill that patient's perceived needs. Beneficence requires that nurses take active, positive steps to help others; it is considered an ethical duty, not merely an act of kindness. Beneficence not only confers benefits; it actively prevents and removes harm. It does not involve acts of good that could result in harm.

As important as the duty to do good and prevent harm, is the duty to weigh the potential good against the potential harm of an action

(Beauchamp & Childress, 1983). Weighing possible benefits and possible harm and determining the extent of each is called utility. (Utility is treated in greater detail in the next part of this chapter.) *Ethical utility* assumes that people have a moral obligation to weigh and balance possible benefits against possible harm in order to maximize benefits and minimize harms. Cost-benefit analysis and risk analysis both attempt to quantify utility. For example, certain medical technologies and medication regimens can have both negative side effects and positive outcomes for patients, especially elderly patients. In the past elderly patients were often restrained in institutional settings to prevent falls and injury. Although intended to prevent harm, mechanical restraint actually contributed to increased morbidity and mortality among elderly patients by causing nerve injury, new onset pressure ulcers, pneumonia, incontinence, increased confusion, and strangulation or asphyxiation. In this case the benefits of restraint do not seem to outweigh the costs or negative outcomes.

Paternalism, or taking the role of knowing what is best for another person, has an implicit dilemma. In assuming a paternal role, the health care provider diminishes the patient's autonomy. Even though the goal is the well-being of the patient, the patient suffers. Do the benefits justify the suffering? Views about whether paternalism is justified differ. Some argue, for example, that physicians or nurses are justified in interfering with a person's intended course of action if that interference protects the person against his or her unreasonably risky choices or actions, such as declining skilled home care when it is needed. Others argue that such paternalism is not justified because it violates the individual's rights and excessively restricts free choice. They argue that the autonomous person can determine his of her best interests more competently than anyone else can (Beauchamp & Childress, 1983).

Describe conflicts you have experienced that involved the principle of beneficence. In what situations would the duty of beneficence cause dilemmas?

Nonmaleficence is the duty to do no harm. Health care delivery rests upon the principle of nonmaleficence because health care providers have the duty not to inflict harm or injure patients. Kapp (1987) expands this definition by stating that nonmaleficence is the principal that, even in those situations in which a particular individual cannot be helped, at least that person should not be harmed.

Nonmaleficence encompasses not only actual harm but risk of harm. Conflicts arise over the degree of harm permissible to risk. Risk of harm is allowed under numerous conditions (e.g., surgical, diagnostic, and therapeutic procedures). A standard of "due care" is recognized both in ethics and in law in which the risk of harm taken is judged against what risk a "reasonable person" would also take. "Due care" is met when the goals are important enough to justify the risks—both the magnitude of harm and the probability of harm—imposed on others (Beauchamp & Childress, 1983).

A nonmaleficence-autonomy dilemma is common in nursing and medicine. Ethical dilemmas about killing versus letting die have contributed to much debate. Some argue that there is a major difference between patients who ask to be allowed to die under certain conditions (i.e., they have a terminal disease and are well informed about their condition) and the patients who ask to be killed. Others argue that letting die and killing are both morally wrong.

Describe conflicts you have experienced that involved the principle of nonmaleficence.

The principle of *justice* implies fairness and is met when individuals receive what they deserve from another individual or society. Just acts are acts that give people that to which they are entitled. What people can justly claim depends on the contractual agreements they have made and on the obligations society assumes regarding their circumstances. For example, a person who has served in the armed forces can justly claim benefits from the Veterans' Administration. A person with an income falling below the poverty line can claim Medicaid benefits.

Distributive justice refers to the proper distribution of social benefits. For example, distributive justice involves deciding whether money is to be allocated for cancer or arthritis research. Dilemmas involving the principle of justice arise when caregivers are forced to make choices among deserving patients. Valid principles of distributive justice include the following (Beauchamp & Childress, 1983, p. 187):

- To each person an equal share
- To each person according to individual needs

- To each person according to individual effort
- To each person according to societal contribution
- To each person according to merit

Beauchamp and Childress also point out that none of these principles can be assessed independently of particular circumstances.

Justice also involves balancing rights and claims. This balancing is referred to as *comparative justice* and it involves balancing the competing claims of different people and deciding who gets what. Thus, comparative justice is affected by the conditions of others in society. Health care providers use the principle of justice when balancing allocation of resources or deciding whose needs to attend to first. Determining whether a person qualifies for a heart transplant (above others) is an example of comparative justice.

> Do health care providers give the elderly and the young equal weight when balancing justice? What kinds of "just rewards" can the elderly claim?

Recognizing Ethical Dilemmas

Most ethical dilemmas involve conflicts among rights, duties, and obligations. The roles nurses play in the medical community (and the medical hierarchy) contribute to some of the dilemmas nurses experience. As employees, nurses must abide by policies established by others. As employees, nurses have obligations to the institutions and physicians; as professionals, however, they are obligated to their patients. As patient advocates, nurses may experience conflict between professional obligations and patients' rights. They are responsible for primary patient care, but have neither authority to make decisions nor accountability for them. Nurses may have limited or even no input into decisions that they must implement, even when they have valuable information to contribute.

Ethical dilemmas are likely to have several components. A ethical dilemma may exist when

(a) moral claims conflict, and people feel that they both should and should not do something,

   (b)   one situation calls for one set of values, but a morally similar situation calls for different ones, and/or

   (c)   human needs conflict, and people must choose to fulfill one person's needs over another's.

IDENTIFYING ETHICAL DILEMMAS IN DISCHARGE PLANNING

Identifying ethical dilemmas in discharge planning includes an analysis of the roles of each party involved in the process. Health care providers have an obligation to provide patients with information they can use to make informed decisions. A variety of factors and different party perspectives have the potential to create situations involving ethical dilemmas.

Informed Decision Making

The role of the caregiver in discharge planning includes providing the patient with sufficient information to make decisions. This includes information about:

- the expected medical condition upon discharge
- the prognosis
- medical and therapeutic regimens
- alternative care settings
- all risks and benefits that accompany each alternative

Factors Affecting Discharge Planning Dilemmas

While medical ethics upholds the principle of autonomy, patients' functional ability sometimes interferes with their ability to make decisions. Thus, the nurse must ask: What is the capacity of the patient to make decisions? The components of competence require that "the patient possess the reasoning capability necessary to integrate the concrete information with his [or her] personal values" (Zuckerman, 1988, p. 320). Note that most elderly patients are capable of making decisions for themselves. However, some patients are capable of making certain decisions, but incapable of making others. Making decisions for these patients requires careful consideration of what they would want if they were able to make decisions for themselves. A minority of patients are incapable of making any decisions.

Patients have different views and definitions of acceptable lifestyles. Some patients will want to return home even with risk rather than be placed in an alternative care facility. If patients are fully informed and able to weigh the risks and benefits, then the principle of autonomy decrees that they have the right to make such a decision.

The involvement of a third party alters the traditional role of the decision-making process between the provider and patient. Third parties (families, services providing home health care, social services, long-term care facilities, etc.) also have rights when they may have a significant role in providing care to the elder. Third party involvement negates the primacy of autonomy even if the elder is fully capable of making decisions because the provider must consider the rights and interests of others.

The discharge plan has to rely on the dependability of community agencies and families, because the discharge environment is, ultimately, beyond the jurisdiction of hospital control. The Prospective Payment System is another invariable, creating time pressures to discharge patients early, perhaps before an effective plan has been established.

On the bottom line, patients' discharge choices can conflict with the caregiver's recommendations or with institutional or family perspectives.

Perspectives of Each Party in the Discharge Planning Effort

The Patient

Patients may not place the same emphasis on restoration or maintenance of health that caregivers do. But decisions about health care options are ultimately the patient's.

Elders frequently have to convince caregivers that they have the capacity to make decisions. But elders have the same right to determine where to live, with whom to associate, and how to pattern and place their lives as other patients. Hospital environments frequently remove the elder's right to autonomy when obvious physical impairments (frailties, speech difficulties, etc.) are present. None of these problems has anything to do with decision-making ability. However, when patients have the decision-making ability but lack the functional capacity to carry out the plans they have made, their decisions depend on others for completion. Ethical and legal principles that enable patients to make autonomous decisions conflict with the reality of the patients' abilities.

Hospital environments affect patients in other ways. They frequently make patients dependent, although law and ethics are based on independence. Patients' functional status often changes in a hospital environment, thus limiting their options.

The Health Care Provider

The health care provider has a legal and ethical obligation to give patients the information necessary for making sound health care decisions. The provider is also obliged, legally and ethically to respect the decisions patients make. These obligations conflict with one another when:

- a patient's decision conflicts with sound health standards
- having worked to restore health, the provider must accept the patient's decision to assume risks
- the provider has an additional obligation to public welfare and policy
- providers view discharge planning as their medical decision rather than the patients' personal decision
- an institution faces financial pressures from delays in discharge

The involvement of a third party changes the relationship between the provider and the patient. As patient advocate, the provider should take into account that the patient's decisions might have been manipulated or coerced by family or another third party. On the other hand, providers need to maintain a working relationship with community services. Providers may have internal conflict when matching a patient to a service if they feel the match will burden that service. When elders decide to return to their home environments, providers may feel obligated to inform third parties of potential dangers (such as the elder forgetting to turn off the stove).

The Acute-Care Institution

The acute care institution has an obligation to ensure the rights of all patients. This includes an obligation to discharge patients with a safe and adequate plan. The institution also has obligations to regulatory and funding bodies. The foundation for institutional decision making is the utilitarian model, ensuring equal care, concern, and resources for all patients. Thus the interest of one patient may be compromised to serve the interests of all.

The Family

Unless a court ruling has appointed a family member as legal guardian, families have no automatic legal right to be involved in the discharge planning process. The only legal duty of the family is for the spouse to provide financial assistance. Families do have a right to participate if requested by the patient. The health care provider may request family involvement.

If the discharge plan relies on the family to carry out tasks and responsibilities, then the family has a right to be consulted first. A discharge plan that relies on family involvement is not deemed an appropriate plan if it cannot be implemented because of family inability or refusal to carry out the actions the plan dictates.

Community Agencies

Because of the differences between supply and demand, cost constraints, and the contractual nature of community agencies, the agency will likely be selective about which clients it accepts. The agency may not want to accept a client it considers to be a physical risk because of liability issues, and/or clients it views as not complying with the agency's rules. Agency selectivity narrows the provider's care plan options and may be the one reason some patients have to compromise their independence and be placed in an alternative care facility.

SOLVING ETHICAL DILEMMAS

A resolution or approach for standardizing ethical decision making in the health care system derives from the mandate to provide equal care to all. Various approaches have been studied to help providers resolve these dilemmas. The section below compares two ethical problem-solving approaches: the "balancing approach" and the "philosophical approach."

Balancing Party Perspectives

As we described above, each party involved in discharge planning has different interests that can bias its perspective in the decision-making process. Therefore, it is important to examine and balance the different interests before delineating roles in the discharge process. In the "balancing approach," the rights of the patient are paramount. This approach underscores the principles governing the relationship between the patient and the provider. Compromise of principles, cooperation among adversaries, and tolerance of conflicting perspectives are essential to conflict resolution. When balancing party perspectives, the following list should be used as protocols:

1. Recognize the perspectives of each party involved.

2. Respect (implement) the patient's wishes and desires if the patient has decision-making ability. Caregivers may have expertise and advice, but the decision is the patient's.

3. Provide all relevant information needed for decision making.

4. Respect the autonomy of the individual.

5. Recognize the multidisciplinary nature of discharge planning. Because a decision is made by a group, the caregiver may have to compromise some principles.

6. List the options that are actually available to the patient. This list should not include every option imaginable, only those that are actually available to the patient. This way the patient maintains a decision-making role.

7. Recognize that patients have the right to assume risk(s) if they are clearly informed of the risks, understand those risks, have been told about alternatives, and if their risk taking does not pose harm to other third parties.

8. Actively solicit information from the patient and family so that all perspectives are considered.

9. Consult legal services if you are unable to resolve conflicts, but realize that legal decisions usually do not provide answers to discharge dilemmas.

Philosophical Approaches

Utilitarianism seeks "the greatest good for the greatest number." It deems an action morally right if the consequences are good or if performing an action would yield good consequences if every one did it. Utilitarianism weighs the benefits of an action against the negative consequences of that action. When the benefits outweigh the costs, then the greatest good is determined. Utilitarian theory suggests that moral decisions are based solely on the consequences of actions, not on the inherent right or wrong of the actions themselves. Hospitals and communities often use this approach when making decisions about how to provide equitable, appropriate, affordable, and accessible services for individuals.

Formalist theory states that an action is right if it is in accordance with a moral principle or rule, (e.g., "Do unto others as you would have them do to you"), and wrong if it violates such a rule. The consequences of the act do not matter. Features of an act that make it right include such things as truth-telling, promise-keeping, and abstract justice and beneficence. Rules and principles are related to the decision itself, not the consequences. The principles apply to all situations. This approach is often used to judge individual acts.

Egoist theory focuses on whether a health care provider is comfortable with a decision. For example, withholding information may be acceptable according to egoist theory because providing information may make the provider uncomfortable.

Steps for Applying Ethical Principles

Various models have been devised to help providers approach ethical decision making. The essential steps for either a utilitarian or philosophical model are described below.

1. Describe the situational facts: persons involved, histories, proposed plan, setting, alternatives, and consequences of alternatives (Henderson & McConnell, 1988).

2. Determine the decision-making questions (Henderson & McConnell, 1988) and gather additional necessary information. For example, Who is the decision maker (patient, family, physician)? What criteria are used to make the decision (legal, economic, physical condition, social, etc.)? What degree of informed consent is needed? What are the ethical principles and how are they relevant to the situation? (Ethical principles applicable to older individuals include high-quality care, respect, beneficence, autonomy, and justice.)

3. Define the dilemma.

4. Generate possible solutions for the dilemma.

5. Weigh the positive and negative consequences of those solutions.

6. Select the best option and act accordingly.

Now that you have a working definition of ethics, and have gained some knowledge in solving ethical dilemmas, apply that knowledge in recognizing and working through problems.

Refer to the Mrs. Loh case below, develop a discharge plan for Mrs. Loh and justify the plan by (a) listing the situational facts, (b) listing the decision-making questions, and (c) explaining the relevance of the ethical principals applicable to older individuals.

Case Study: *Mrs. Loh*

Mrs. Loh, age 83, is hospitalized as an emergency patient with a broken hip. She apparently fell when getting up from her sewing machine. She lives alone, and has one son who lives in another part of the country. Local family consists of two brothers, their wives, three nieces, and a nephew. One brother believes Mrs. Loh belongs in a nursing home because she is incontinent and seems unable to cope with housekeeping anymore. The brother's wife and Mrs. Loh do not get along. The other brother is seriously impaired with Parkinson's disease. His wife, who works full time in addition to caring for her husband, gets along with Mrs. Loh but has little time available. The niece and nephew, both in their early 50s, are fully occupied with their own lives, and see Mrs. Loh only on holidays.

Mrs. Loh seems well nourished but physically run down; her overall appearance improves with bed rest. From conversations with Mrs. Loh and with her regular doctor, an internist, you learn that she is alert, energetic, has many friends, and leads an active life. She has suffered two small strokes, uses a hearing aid, and had an unsuccessful surgery a few years ago to try to correct the urinary problem. The doctor monitors her blood pressure regularly, which has been good for the past 3 years. The doctor also mentions how good Mrs. Loh always looks when she comes to see him.

Mrs. Loh tells you that she loves to cook, hates to clean, and makes all of her own clothes. She also says that when she leaves the hospital she wants to go home. A neighbor who often sees Mrs. Loh tells you that the apartment is "a mess," that she is trying to deal with the worst of it, but that she doesn't think Mrs. Loh could stay there comfortably while recuperating from her hip surgery.

Mrs. Loh receives a modest monthly income that she describes as "adequate" and belongs to a Medicare-approved HMO.

Questions for Consider

1. What are Mrs. Loh's short-term care needs upon discharge?

2. What options might you consider for meeting those needs?

3. What factors would influence you to recommend particular options?

4. What are Mrs. Loh's long-term care needs?

5. What options might you consider for meeting those needs?

6. What factors influence your decisions?

The Loh case represents a conflict between the ethical principles of autonomy and beneficence. Nurses want to respect the patient's right to make an informed decision about care, but at the same time nurses feel the need to promote good and to prevent harm. Although Mrs. Loh wants to return home and should be allowed to do so, according to the principles of autonomy, a discharge home without adequate support could jeopardize her health. Therefore, discharge plans for Mrs. Loh should consider the least restrictive postdischarge environment that meets Mrs. Loh's custodial and health care needs. Cost is also an important factor to consider here, as Mrs. Loh's Medicare-approved HMO will not cover her custodial care.

SUMMARY

The Key points of the chapter are:

1. Most ethical dilemmas involve conflicts among rights, duties, and obligations.
2. Health care providers have an obligation to help the patient make an informed decision.
3. The parties involved in discharge planning have different interests that can bias their perspective in the decision-making process. Therefore, it is important to examine and balance the different party interests before delineating roles in discharge planning.
4. Ethical decision making often involves weighing the positive and negative consequences of various actions for the patient and others involved in the discharge plan.

CLINICAL EXERCISE

Identify one ethical issue faced in a discharge planning case at your institution and document what was done.

REFERENCES

American Nurses Association. (1976). *Code for nurses with interpretive statements*. Kansas City, MO: American Nurses Association.

Aroskar, M. A. (1980). Anatomy of an ethical dilemma: The theory. *American Journal of Nursing, 80*, 658–660.

Beauchamp, T. L., & Childress, J. F. (1983). *Principles of biomedical ethics* (2nd ed.). New York: Oxford University Press.

Henderson, M. L., & McConnell, E. S. (1988). Ethical considerations. In M. A. Matteson & E. S. McConnell (Eds.), *Gerontological nursing: Concepts and practice* (pp. 93–121). Philadelphia: Saunders.

Kapp, M. (1987). Interprofessional relationships in geriatrics: Ethical and legal considerations. *Gerontologist, 27,* 547–552.

Strumpf, N. E., & Paier, G. (1992). Ethical issues. In T. T. Fulmer & M. K. Walker (Eds.), *Critical care nursing of the elderly* (pp. 296–305). New York: Springer.

Zuckerman, C. (1988). Ethical and legal issues. In P. J. Volland (Ed.), *Discharge planning: An interdisciplinary approach to continuity of care* (pp. 317–336). Owings Mill, MD: National Health Publishing.

SUGGESTED READINGS

Callahan, D. (1987). *Setting limits.* New York: Simon & Schuster.

Lynn, J. (1988). Conflicts of interest in medical decision making. *Journal of the American Geriatrics Society, 36,* 945–950.

Post, S. (1989). Biomedical ethics and the elderly: An emerging focus. *Gerontologist, 29,* 568–570.

Chapter **8**

MONITORING AND EVALUATING DISCHARGE PLANS

LEARNING OBJECTIVES

At the end of this chapter, readers will be able to:

1. Discuss the history and development of quality assurance
2. Define quality assurance
3. Relate the principles of quality assurance to discharge planning at their home institutions
4. Recognize standards by which quality of care is measured
5. Monitor the quality of the discharge planning process within the acute care setting

Monitoring and evaluating discharge plans are important because of discharge planning's potential for reducing readmissions and its evaluation of the possibility of meeting continuing care needs in alternative, less costly levels of care (Conte, 1983). In designing, documenting, and evaluating discharge plans, nurses play a crucial and pivotal role. They are often aware of the patient's functional, physical, and cognitive abilities and how these will affect and determine patient functioning after discharge. This chapter provides nurses with basic information about quality assurance and standards of care. In addition, nurses examine ways that quality assurance relates specifically to discharge planning and design plans for monitoring and evaluating discharge plans for patients in their care.

The chapter begins with an introduction to quality assurance. Definitions and perceptions of quality as they relate to health care and to other areas of life are described. The origins of quality assurance (QA) and a working definition for QA are discussed.

A case study is presented so that readers can examine ways they might improve the quality of care for the case study. This is followed by material on the relationship between QA and discharge planning that focuses on the role of the physician review organizations (PROs) and examines their approach to reviewing a case where quality care is in question.

Four case studies are presented for practice in delineating the major discharge planning and quality assurance issues.

A discussion of "standards of care" as they relate to quality assurance follows. This illustrates the "standard of care" concept by using examples of standards and discussing approaches to developing these standards.

At the end of the chapter readers complete Part IV of their action plan for improving discharge planning at their institutions. In this activity readers outline the obstacles they expect to encounter in implementing their action plan and the potential solutions for overcoming these obstacles.

AN INTRODUCTION TO QUALITY ASSURANCE

Defining Quality of Care

What do we mean by quality? Definitions vary. Quality may be one's own definitions of personal excellence. Often quality is used in reference to something else, for example, a quality product, quality care, quality time. In these cases "quality" indicates something good and valued, durable and lasting. Yet, quality to one person may not be quality to another and for this reason, individuals have tried to quantify and operationalize what we mean when we talk about quality. Researchers and policy makers, for example, have tried to standardize what is meant by quality of life and quality care. In this respect, quality becomes a standard established by groups, institutions, or other individuals.

The definition of quality in health care has changed over time. With the introduction of the Prospective Payment System, for example, physician review organizations (PROs) began to focus on quality-of-care issues to ensure that quality would not be compromised by premature discharge. Thus, PROs would meet prospective payment regulations and would be able to receive funding or Medicare reimbursement. In the early 1980s, the Department of Health and Human Services began contracting with physician review organizations to perform quality control over peer review.

History and Development of Quality Assurance

Health care providers historically have been concerned with the maintenance and improvement of quality of care for hospitalized patients. As early as 1860 individuals were trying to ensure that quality care was provided to patients. But it was not until 1965, with the passage of the Medicare and Medicaid acts, that quality assurance developed into a science of its own. Quality assurance is still in its infancy. Health care providers are just learning to develop tools to evaluate the quality and appropriateness of care rendered to patients at their institutions. A brief history of QA is outlined in Table 8.1.

The Principles of Quality Assurance

Quality assurance today involves the process of monitoring and evaluating the quality and appropriateness of care. It is also a process that:

- Focuses on the outcomes of patient care
- Employs monitoring and evaluation methods to determine quality and appropriateness of patient planning and care
- Investigates the structure, process, and outcome components of care provided
- Seeks to identify deficiencies in care provided and plans interventions to improve care
- Focuses on identifying appropriate or inappropriate patterns of care within and across hospitals, but also conducts individual case reviews when necessary
- Identifies ways health care providers can improve their delivery of care

TABLE 8.1   The Evolution of Quality Assurance

1860s	Florence Nightingale collected hospital statistics to assess nursing care provided to casualties of the American Civil War. (Rehr, 1979)
Early 1900s	Dr. Richard Cabot at Massachusetts General Hospital attempted to uncover errors by comparing autopsy results with information in medical records. Dr. Ernest Codman reviewed outcome data (and results) on all of his surgical patients. (Jacobs, Christoffel, & Dixon, 1976)
1951	Joint Commissions on the Accreditation of Hospitals (JACH) setting standards.
1952	JCAH began surveying hospitals. Focus was on an efficient fiscal plant, qualified personnel, and properly developed procedures.
1950s & 1960s	Internal hospital committees evaluated care through retrospective audits. These activities were only conducted in about 20% of hospitals nationwide. Amendments to the Social Security Act mandated that quality assurance programs be implemented in every hospital. JCAH revised accreditation standards requiring review of admission necessity, lengths of stay, discharge practices, and services ordered and provided.
1970	JCAH adopted MCEs (Medical Care Evaluation concept).
1972	Medicare and JCAH both required: • Utilization review of necessity of admission, duration of stay, and professional services furnished • Medical care evaluations JCAH introduced PEP (Performance Evaluation Procedure) PEP was a methodology for insuring quality of care: • Identify deficiencies • Implement actions to eliminate problems • Evaluated patient outcomes against criteria • Focused on outcome • Process review undertaken when outcome was poor Public Law 92–603 passed. • Established PSROs (Professional Standard Review Organizations), which focused on cost control. • Purpose was to ensure that health services were necessary, met standards of care, and were provided economically.

TABLE 8.1 *Continued*

	• Emphasis was on peer review and audits of the medical profession.
1980	JCAH mandated hospitals to focus QA attention on problem areas. • QA to focus on identifying, assessing, and resolving known or suspect problems in patient care. • Application was to be prospective, concurrent, or retrospective. • All health professionals now required to perform QA. • All health professionals now required to engage in peer review.
1982	Tax Equity and Fiscal Responsibility (TEFRA) established the Prospective Payment System (PPS) for Medicare. • Uses the diagnosis-related groups (DRGs)-based reimbursement system. • Focus of PPS is on cost containment: — Uses DRGs to determine reimbursement by category. — Hospital gains if patient is discharged early, suffers losses if patient's stay exceeds DRG allocation of days. • PROs (Peer Review Organizations) focused on quality of care issues, attempts to ensure quality will not be compromised by premature discharge, etc. in order to meet PPS regulations and receive funding. • Department of Health and Human Services began contracting with physician review organizations (PROs) to perform utilization review and quality control over peer review.

Note. Adapted from B. Berkman, 1988, "Quality assurance, utilization review, and discharge planning," by B. Berkman, in P.J. Volland (Ed.), *Discharge planning: An interdisciplinary approach to continuity of care* (pp. 255–277), 1988, Owings Mills, MD: National Health Publishing.

Refer to the Ms. Monroe case below*. Apply the principles of quality assurance defined above. Think about ways Ms. Monroe's quality of care is compromised and ways you might assure or improve her quality of care.

* This case was adapted from one originally developed by Nancy Miller, RN, MS.

Case Study: *Ms. Monroe*

Ms. Monroe is an 80-year-old white female with a history of hypertension, a cerebrovascular accident with mild right residual hemiparesis, and degenerative joint disease. She was found by neighbors in her apartment after a fall and brought by EMTs to the emergency unit. She complained of urinary urgency and frequency, and was febrile on admission. Ms. Monroe was diagnosed with a left pneumonia and a urinary tract infection, which were both treated with antibiotics during her hospitalization. She also received physical therapy to improve her strength and help her adjust to using a walker.

Ms. Monroe lives alone in an elderly housing complex and has no available family for support. The bathroom in her apartment is equipped with a tub seat and safety rails, but she needs assistance with bathing and dressing. It was noted at admission that she did not dress fully every day. However, Ms. Monroe can cook her own meals.

Ms. Monroe will be discharged to her home with requests for (a) skilled nursing care twice a week to monitor medications, (b) home health aide 5 times a week, 4–6 hours per day to assist with bathing and dressing, and (c) physical therapy 3 times a week to establish gait stability and safety.

Ms. Monroe is typical of the patients you see in the acute care setting. She is at risk of falling in the home and of readmission. For this reason you want to assure that Ms. Monroe and others like her receive quality care and that the discharge planning process ensures that quality.

Questions to Consider

1.   Is the discharge planning process appropriate? Appropriateness means the extent to which the treatment is effective, indicated, or needed. Patient needs and wants should always be a priority. The treatment is only appropriate if it is what the patient wants. Does Ms. Monroe agree with her plan?

2.   Will the discharge plan result in improved health and quality of life for the patient? Are the results what you expected? Will the patient be discharged home or to an institution? Did the patient develop coping strategies to deal with functional disabilities?

3.   Were there any treatments or procedures implemented that improved patient compliance with medication or therapy regimens? Did these regimens improve functional ability? Did they make the patient feel more independent?

4.   How might you measure the effectiveness of Ms. Monroe's plan or other discharge plans? How were the changes made? What processes or procedures were the most effective in improving, for example, patient independence or functional ability? How and why were they effective? What was the result of these procedures?

5.   What deficiencies exist and how might you eliminate these?

6.   Is Ms. Monroe receiving quality care? Does she exemplify others?

7.   How does my delivery of care affect the overall quality of care at my home institution?

QUALITY ASSURANCE AND DISCHARGE PLANNING

Economic incentives to restrict resource use fostered new concerns about premature discharge and resulting costly readmissions. As noted earlier, discharge planning became important because of its potential to reduce readmissions and evaluate the possibility of meeting continuing care needs in alternative, less costly levels of care. Nurses need to ensure that patients receive adequate and appropriate care while in the hospital and leave hospitals with adequate follow-up care. This way they can help reduce premature discharge at their institutions and help assure that patient discharge plans are adequate to meet the needs of the patient and prevent unnecessary readmissions.

Peer Review Organizations and Discharge Planning

The Tax Equity and Fiscal Responsibility Act (TEFRA) established the Prospective Payment System for Medicare with reimbursement based on its diagnostic-related groups. The TEFRA legislation also created the Peer Improvement Act in which the Department of Health and Human Services enters into agreements with physician review organizations (PROs) to perform utilization review and quality control over peer review.

The PROs emphasize quality-of-care issues more than cost control. They ensure that Medicare pays only for services that are medically reasonable and necessary, that these services meet professionally recognized high-quality standards; and that services are provided in the most cost-effective way (Berkman, 1988). In particular, their goals, discussed below, are:

1. Reduce premature discharge and thus, high-risk readmissions.
2. Ensure that patients get the services they need.
3. Prevent overutilization or manipulation of other services.

To determine whether a premature discharge was involved, quality assurance focuses on the cause of the readmission. The Health Care Financing Administration (HCFA) defines a premature discharge as one in which the patient is not medically stable and where there is a continuing need for acute inpatient care (American Hospital Association, 1986). HCFAs generic criteria for medical stability include:

- Acceptable blood pressure ranges on the day before or the day of discharge
- Acceptable temperature ranges on the day before or the day of discharge
- No abnormal test results, not otherwise explained in the record
- No IV fluids or drugs on the day of discharge (with appropriate exceptions)
- No abnormal drainage from surgical wounds

The PRO may use additional criteria. The PRO will usually review a case if it fails one or more generic screens. A physician reviewer is assigned the case and must then determine whether the staff implemented a proper discharge plan.

Patients should not be denied services because of hospitals goals to meet discharge deadlines. If the physician reviewer finds that necessary discharge procedures were lacking or that the patient was denied necessary services, then the hospital may be denied payment. As Lazar (1983) explains, the PROs will attempt to reduce unnecessary readmissions that result from inadequate medical care in a prior admission or from inadequate discharge planning.

Other services must not be overutilized or manipulated in order to avoid incurring in-house debt (such as transfers to other hospitals). Hospitals are not only concerned about potential loss of revenue if patients stay too long, but they also wish to avoid premature discharge. Thus, the discharge planning process must focus on strong utilization management techniques (Granatir, 1985).

The Quality Assurance Approach

The quality assurance approach is known by many names. These include (Berkman, 1988) *audit, monitoring system, patient care evaluation, social health care evaluation, performance evaluation procedure, health services review organization audit,* and *medical care evaluation.*

Two models commonly used in evaluating discharge planning include the American Nurses Association's (ANA) and the Joint Commissions on Accreditation of Hospitals' (JCAH) models. The ANA five-step model uses the following steps:

1. Design the study.
2. Establish the criteria.
3. Gather the data.
4. Interpret the data.
5. Take action.

The JCAH follows these steps:

1. Assign responsibility.
2. Delineate scope of care.
3. Identify important aspects of care.
4. Identify indicators related to these aspects of care.
5. Establish thresholds for evaluation related to the indicators.
6. Collect and organize data.
7. Evaluate care when thresholds are reached.
8. Take actions to improve care.
9. Assess the effectiveness of the actions and document improvement.
10. Communicate relevant information to the organization-wide quality assurance programs.

A quality assurance program that studies the quality and appropriateness of discharge planning will, generally, look for the presence of discharge planning, and a standardized documentation format for recording the discharge plan. It will require evidence of a patient's understanding of the discharge plan and of discharge instructions. There must be evidence of multidisciplinary involvement. The feasibility of the post-hospital plan primarily determines its appropriateness.

Note that effective and thorough documentation will assist in monitoring discharge planning at your institution. When and if you decide to study a particular problem, stringent documentation practices may prove helpful. A hospital's recording system should enable the collection of data in an orderly fashion. (Refer to Appendix A and B of this chapter for copies of quality assurance instruments used by nursing and social service department staff at the Beth Israel Hospital in Boston, MA.) Most often, the medical record has been the primary source of documentation in the hospital. However, one of the major drawbacks of the medical record system is that it is not standardized for uniform entry. Records are sometimes poorly organized and entries are uneven in amount of detail. For this reason, many are moving toward computerized data systems (see Pinchbeck & Span, 1984; and Fagan, 1984).

Concentrating our efforts on developing discharge plans that work should lessen the incidence of readmission because of poor planning for care outside of the hospital environment. Thus, as mentioned above, discharge planning becomes a major focus for maintaining the quality of patient care. Effective discharge planning should decrease the potential for readmission, identify economic and appropriate care alternatives, and increase patient satisfaction.

Refer to the cases below and consider them in the light of quality assurance criteria.* Ask yourself:

1. Is the patient at risk for readmission?
2. Was the patient medically stable at discharge?
3. Did the patient agree with the discharge plan?
4. Was documentation of the plan thorough?

---

* These cases were adapted from ones originally developed by Nancy Miller, RN, MS.

Case Study 1: *Ms. Holland*

Ms. Holland, an 80-year-old woman, was discharged from the hospital to the care of her niece. The niece lives close to Ms. Holland and occasionally stops by to check on her. Ms. Holland's niece claimed that she would be able to arrange for all her aunt's health care needs and would contact the necessary service agencies. The attending nurse had already outlined an intricate discharge plan that included a list of needed and available services and agreed to give the list to the niece and let her make the connections.

Shortly after discharge, Ms. Holland suffered a fall in her home and sustained a minor injury. She filed a compliant with the hospital claiming that she received no services or assistance, and that their absence contributed to her fall. It turns out that Ms. Holland's niece failed to connect her aunt with the needed services.

Major Question: Should Ms. Holland's niece have been trusted to connect her with the needed services? Does this indicate the need for a new protocol?
Issues: Patient satisfaction, readmission, patient agreement with plan.

Case Study 2: *Mr. Alvarez*

Mr. Alvarez's admitting diagnosis was failure to thrive. After a short stay in the hospital, this 82-year-old man was discharged to a nearby nursing home. Within 3 days Mr. Alvarez was back in the hospital.

His case was called before the peer review organization, which found that he had a temperature of 101°F 24 hours prior to discharge. Moreover, the PRO was unable to find any vital signs listed in the patient's medical record. The person monitoring the patient was not recording the necessary data thoroughly.

Major Question: Was this a premature discharge?
Issues: Medical stability, proper documentation, standards of care.

Case Study 3: *Mr. Navarro*

Mr. Navarro is an 65-year-old man who was admitted after suffering a mild stroke. When he was discharged home, Mr. Navarro required much assistance with his activities of daily living. Therefore, he was matched with homemaker services and a home health aide who came into his home for 4 hours per day and 2 hours per day respectively.

A few weeks later, hospital staff telephoned Mr. Navarro to determine whether the services were appropriate. Mr. Navarro complained vigorously and said that the services were not meeting his needs and were inadequate.

Major Question: How do you determine whether the services were appropriate?

Issues: Patients' perceptions of appropriate care, follow-up procedures, patient satisfaction, balancing patient needs with costs.

Case Study 4: *Mrs. Robertson*

Mrs. Robertson is a 75-year-old woman with a history of diabetes and degenerative joint disease. She was originally admitted to the hospital for complications resulting from her diabetes. She reported that she lives down the street from her daughter, who stops in often and assists her with her household duties.

Upon discharge, her primary nurse realized that Mrs. Robertson might need additional assistance in the home with her cooking, cleaning, bathing, and other activities. When the daughter was asked about her availability to help her mother with the additional tasks of dressing and bathing, the daughter said that she did not want this responsibility. Therefore, the nurse made arrangements to have a homemaker visit Mrs. Robertson 4 days a week for 4 hours a day.

Major Question: Is this the most effective discharge plan?

Issues: Costs, appropriateness of care, patient satisfaction, balancing patient and caregiver needs.

ESTABLISHING STANDARDS OF CARE

Standards are the criteria by which we measure quality of care. According to Berkman (1988, p. 264) standards "are value judgments explicitly stated and arrived at by professionals to determine that similar situations can be recognized and similarly judged . . . [standards] must be stated in measurable not descriptive terms and must be precise enough to permit accurate evaluation."

Three different types of criteria are used for evaluating practice (Donabedian, 1969). These include structure, process, and outcomes. *Structure* refers to the setting in which care is delivered: dynamics within the care setting, variations within care-provider groups, and interactions among care providers (Jennings, 1991). *Process* refers to the steps one performs when carrying out an activity. For nurses, these steps fall into two categories: systems of nursing and multidisciplinary processes. Discharge planning spans both of these categories (Closs & Tierney, 1993). *Outcomes* refers—in the case of discharge planning—to positive outcomes associated with the patient, the family, and cost of care (Naylor, 1990). For example, patient outcomes have been evaluated in terms of length of stay, satisfaction with discharge arrangements, frequency of postdischarge problems and rehospitalization, and satisfaction with postdischarge services and support. Research has tended to concentrate on outcomes of health care rather than the structure and process of health care (Thomas & Bond, 1991).

As Closs and Tierney (1993) note, there are certain conceptual difficulties in the isolation or integration of structure, process, and outcomes. It is often difficult to decide which of these three categories best defines a particular aspect of nursing care. Some examples of structure, process, and outcome standards follow:

1. *Area Agency on Aging (AAA) process standard:* The coordination of discharge planning must integrate teaching about physical care to facilitate appropriate self-care in the home.

2. *Joint Commissions on the Accreditation of Hospitals (JCAH) process standard:* Patients who are discharged from the hospital requiring nursing care should receive instructions and individualized counseling prior to discharge.

3. *Massachusetts Physician Review Organizations (Mass PRO) structure standard:* Adequacy of discharge planning is measured by the

presence of a discharge planning intervention prior to discharge and a documented plan for appropriate follow-up care.

4. *Massachusetts Department of Public Health structure standard:* The discharge plan shall include, at a minimum, (a) the service arranged for the patient, (b) the names, addresses, and telephone numbers of service providers, (c) the service schedule as requested by the hospital, (d) medications prescribed and instructions for their use or verification that such information was provided separately, and (e) scheduled follow-up medical appointments or verification that such information was provided separately.

5. *Nursing service process standard:* Comprehensive assessment of the patient includes sociodemographics, physical and mental status, functional status, family and community resources, and patient family values and preferences.

6. *Nursing service outcome standard:* After discharge, patients and their families are assisted by support systems necessary to provide for the patients' posthospital care.

Developing Standards

There are generally two accepted approaches to developing standards (Berkman, 1988). First, studies of practice are surveyed.

Usually the included studies have gathered large quantities of normative data describing practice. Statistical ranges are then calculated from these norms which become the accepted standard. Second, expert judges, selected from hospital professionals, review written case material or observe practice, reach consensus, and set acceptable standards of care. These judges must reach agreement on protocols for "good care" and "good practice" in a given situation based not on examining patient records or direct observation, but on practice wisdom.

DESIGNING A QUALITY ASSURANCE STUDY

The American Nurses Association (ANA; 1975) model, described earlier in this chapter, points out how one designs a quality assurance study and develops a monitor. You may use the JCAH model if you feel more comfortable with that one. However, this book attempts to mesh elements of both models in the description below.

Designing the Study

To conduct a quality assurance study you must first select a topic. What is the major aspect of discharge planning that you want to study or evaluate? Choose from problems you know or suspect exist. Problems can be discerned from a review of such things as patient questionnaires, incident reports, previous quality assurance studies, surveys, and observation.

Next, select relevant nursing standard you need to ensure are being implemented. Standards can be selected from such things as professional standards of practice, standards set by accrediting bodies, and standardized documentation protocols. Documentation, for example, helps determine the appropriateness and effectiveness of a plan, and the understanding and satisfaction of the patient with the plan. The JCAH *Accreditation Manual for Hospitals* (1987) has described the role of nurses in documenting issues relevant to discharge planning as follows:

- NR. 5.6: Documentation of nursing care is pertinent and concise and reflects patient status.
- NR. 5.6.4: As appropriate, patients who are discharged from the hospital and require nursing care receive instructions and individualized counseling prior to discharge.
- NR. 5.6.4.1: Evidence of the instructions and the patient's family's understanding of these instructions is noted in the patient's medical record.
- NR. 5.6.4.2: Such instructions and counseling are consistent with the responsible medical practitioner's instructions.

Then, set the specifications of the project. What patient population will be studied? Who are the health care providers for that population? When will the criteria be set and who will be involved in the process? When will the data be gathered and who will do it? Is approval needed prior to collection? Are there any deadlines (such as those superimposed by external review boards)? Are any unusual or excessive costs involved in the study?

Establishing the Criteria or Indicators

First, decide if yours *is a process, structure, or outcome review*. You may begin a study using criteria and indicators that have already been established, but whether standard or original, they must be valid and measurable. Validity can be established by showing testimony of expert consultants; literature demonstrating protocols and data; regulatory policy; standards of nursing, department, and/or institution; or results of your own clinical research. Measurable terms include behavioral descriptions, operational definitions, numerical values, time, and statements of expected outcome.

Establish thresholds for evaluation by including statements as to whether or not you expect 100% compliance to the criteria and, if not, what the expectations would be.

Gathering the Data

Plan how to gather the data. Are the indicators and criteria appropriate for the data source?

You may need to add data-gathering instructions to the criteria. Determine what tools and sources of information will be used. Identify what additional information will be gathered to help the analysis process. Finalize the study population and describe sampling procedures (e.g., 5 patients per day, per unit). Conduct a pilot study to determine appropriateness and effectiveness of data-gathering tools before implementing the larger scale study.

Display the data as forms or graphs; data should clearly state the criteria and show compliance in terms of frequency and percentages. Interpret data by adding explanations of samplings, findings, justifiable variations, and other correlations. Check the effectiveness of the display by asking another nurse to look at and interpret the data out loud. If the interpretation is correct then you can assume your display relates the information you intend it to.

Interpreting the Data

Is care compliant with the standard? Identify strengths and weaknesses in the program being evaluated. Determine how much of a deficiency is acceptable, and to what degree a deficiency can actually be improved.

In reviewing your work, re-examine the data to ascertain that no errors were committed in the data-gathering process. Keep a record of hunches, calculations, and other data. This is the stage at which to draw conclusions, set priorities, choose critical areas to study and act on, try to visually reconstruct the sequence of events that may have led to the deficiency, determine whether or not strengths and deficiencies are related in any way (e.g., one unit only, only the elderly, one shift only).

Categorize the deficiency to help guide action. Problems in the areas of knowledge, performance, motivation, supervision, communication, resources, planning, and documentation will all require different types of response.

Taking Action

What actions can one take to ensure that care is compliant with the standard? Posting results is a first step in correcting deficiencies.

At the same time, propose actions for each category of deficiency. Select a plan. Before starting, re-examine to be certain you have identified the real problem. Then begin implementation of your plan.

If follow-up involves depending on others to implement the plan or is outside of your authority, you can still see the project through by maintaining contact with the people involved. Follow-up involves monitoring the actions taken, as well as results, keeping a record, and reviewing tasks. Follow-up may also necessitate applying sanctions for unmet deadlines, such as revising assignments. It may be necessary to repeat the study, develop a continuous monitor, and/or invite other disciplines to participate.

As with other nursing processes, quality assurance is subject to evaluation. In evaluating the study's effectiveness you need to determine if it met its goals. In evaluating its efficiency you need to determine if it ran smoothly.

Developing Action Plans to Improve Discharge Planning: Part IV

Complete Part IV of your action plan to improve discharge planning at your home institution. (See p. 199 for a copy of the Part IV Worksheet.)

In Part IV of the action plan you will anticipate the potential obstacles to implementing the plan and outline solutions to those obstacles. Suppose, for example, that you believe your plan to implement a new preadmission screening tool will not work, because nurse and hospital administrators may be reluctant to approve the new instrument. One way to overcome this obstacle is to involve nurse and other hospital administrators from the beginning of the plan, and include them at every stage of the process. If the administration still refuses, you might consider an alternative strategy to improving patient outcomes postdischarge and reducing readmissions. You might also consider mustering staff support and approaching the administration again.

SUMMARY

The key points of the chapter are:

1.   With the introduction of the Prospective Payment System, PROs began to focus on quality of care to ensure that quality would not be compromised by premature discharge.

2.   Discharge planning became important because of the potential for reducing readmissions and the possibility of meeting continuing care needs with alternative, less costly levels of care.

3.   Nurses play a crucial role in evaluating and monitoring discharge plans since they are aware of the patient's functional, physical, and cognitive abilities and how these will affect and determine patient functioning after discharge.

4.   Nurses can help reduce premature discharge and prevent unnecessary readmissions by ensuring that patients receive adequate and appropriate care while in the hospital and that they leave the hospital with adequate follow-up care.

5.   Standards are criteria by which nurses can measure quality of care. As such, these standards should be stated in measurable terms rather than descriptive terms, and should be precise enough to permit accurate evaluation.

CLINICAL EXERCISE

Monitor the quality assurance specialist or individual who assumes the duties of monitoring quality care at your institution. Then write a short description of the quality assurance system in place. If you wish to pursue the issue further, design a quality assurance study or monitor the quality of care for a particular patient or for a particular aspect of care at your institution.

REFERENCES

American Hospital Association. (1986). *Issue brief: Discharge review by PROs*. Washington, DC: American Hospital Association.

American Nurses Association. (1975). *Continuity of care and discharge planning programs in institutions and community agencies*. (Publications Code NP-49). Kansas City: Author.

Berkman, B. (1988). Quality assurance, utilization review, and discharge planning. In P. J. Volland (Ed.), *Discharge planning: An interdisciplinary approach to continuity of care* (pp. 255–277). Owings Mills, MD: National Health Publishing.

Closs, S. J., & Tierney, A. J. (1993). The complexities of using a structure, process, and outcome framework: The case of an evaluation of discharge planning for elderly patients. *Journal of Advanced Nursing, 18*, 1279–1287.

Conte, M. A. (1983). PSRO nursing perspective. In *Diagnosis-related groups: The effect in New Jersey, the potential for the nation* (pp. 151–154). Washington, DC: U. S. Department of Health and Human Services, Health Care Financing Administration.

Donabedian, A. (1969). Quality of care: Problems of measurement. Part II: Some issues of evaluating the quality of nursing care. *American Journal of Public Health, 59*, 1833–1836.

Fagan, J. (1984). Developing an information system for discharge planning under prospective pricing. *Discharge Planning Update, 4*, 5–8.

Granatir, T. (1985). Peer review organizations: Implications for discharge planning. *Discharge Planning Update, 5*(3), 4–10.

Jennings, B. M. (1991). Patient outcomes research: Seizing the opportunity. *Advances in Nursing Science, 14*(2), 59–72.

Joint Commission on Accreditation of Hospitals. (1987). *Accreditation manual for hospitals*. Chicago: Author.

Lazar, A. (1983). Utilization review organizations' roles under Medicare's Prospective Payment System. In *Diagnosis-related groups: The effect in New Jersey, the potential for the nation* (pp. 163–64). Washington, DC: Department of Health and Human Services, Health Care Financing Administration.

Naylor, M. D. (1990). Comprehensive discharge planning for the elderly. *Research in Nursing and Health, 13,* 327–347.

Pinchbeck, B., & Span, A. (1984). *How to develop a computer information system for discharge planning departments.* Beaver, PA: Medical Center of Beaver County.

Thomas, L. H., & Bond, S. (1991). Outcomes of nursing care: The case of primary nursing. *International Journal of Nursing Studies, 28*(4), 291–314.

SUGGESTED READINGS

Beckman, J. S. (1987). What is a standard of practice? *Journal of Nursing Quality Assurance, 1*(2), 1–6.

DeVet, C. (Ed.). (1987). *The monitoring source book.* Chicago: Core Communications.

Esper, P. S. (1988). Discharge planning: A quality assurance approach. *Nursing Management, 19*(10), 66–68.

Miesenheimer, C. G. (Ed.) (1985). *Quality assurance: A complete guide to effective programs.* Rockville, MD: Aspen.

Nice, A. (1989). Multidisciplinary discharge screen. *Journal of Nursing Quality Assurance, 3*(2): 63–68.

Smeltzer, C. H., Hinshaw, A. S., & Feltman, B. (1987). The benefits of staff nurse involvement in monitoring the quality of patient care. *Journal of Nursing Quality Assurance, 1*(3), 1–7.

Whittaker, A., & McCanless, L. (1988). Nursing peer review: Monitoring the appropriateness and outcome of nursing care. *Journal of Nursing Quality Assurance, 2*(2), 24–31.

APPENDIX A

Continuing Care Documentation Audit Criteria

Code _____   Date _____

Unit _____   Rater _____

Key: C = Complete   A = Absent

       I = Incomplete   NA = Not Applicable

Assessment

Does nursing admission include notation of the following FHPA's?

	C	I	A	NA	Comments
1. Health perception–health management pattern:					
a. General health status					
b. Self-care practices					
c. Health behaviors					
2. Nutritional-Metabolic pattern:					
a. Appetite/daily intake					
b. Weight loss/gain					
c. Dental status (dentures)					
d. Skin condition					
e. Temperature					
3. Elimination pattern					
a. Bowel elimination pattern					
b. Urinary elimination pattern					

4. Activity-exercise pattern:

a. P, R, BP

b. Assistive devices

c. Perceived ability for (please check)

feeding ——— bathing ——— toiletting ——— bed mobility ——— dressing ——— grooming ———

general mobility ——— meal preparation ——— home maintenance ——— shopping ——— transportation ———

5. Sleep-rest pattern:

a. Sleep onset problems

b. Rest periods

c. Aids (med., music)

6. Cognitive-perceptual pattern:

a. Hearing difficulty (hearing aid)

b. Visual difficulty (eyeglasses)

c. Signs and symptoms of pain

d. Pain management

e. Intellect (i.e., memory, orientation,

recognition,

calculation)

7. Self-perception–self-concept pattern:									
a. Emotional state (affect or mood, self-esteem)									
b. Behavior clues– dress, appropriateness, attentiveness									
8. Roles-relationship pattern:									
a. Family structure/significant others (include any role conflicts)									
b. Living situation (living alone, neighborhood)									
c. Dependent or independent/self care									
9. Sexuality-reproductive pattern:									
a. Sexual relations (problems, changes)									
b. Birth control measures									
c. OB/GYN History (i.e., menses, L&D status)									
10. Coping-stress tolerance pattern:									
a. Recent changes in life/lifestyle									
b. Coping mechanisms (i.e., sharing med., ETOH, drugs)									

11. Value-belief pattern:

   a. Religious background/practices

   b. Ethnic and cultural norms/mores

PLAN

Does the nursing administration assessment include notation of the following?

1. Previous service provided by—

   a. Visiting Nurse Association

   b. Home health agency

   c. Home care program

   d. Homemaker/home health care aide

   e. Other community support service (i.e., hospice, Adult Day Care, FISH, Meals on Wheels, AAA, etc.)

   f. Physician

2. Nursing Home Resident

3. Initial goal/plan for discharge

a. Home

b. Home with supports

c. Alternative care facility

d. Other

IMPLEMENTATION

Has collaboration (intervention by the following health team members) been documented in the patient record?

1. Nursing (i.e., PN, AN, nurse specialists)

2. Medicine

3. Social Services

4. Physical medicine (i.e., PT, OR, RT (speech)

5. Nutritionists

Does the nursing care plan include documantation of updated discharge plans?

EVALUATION

1. Does the medical record include either

a. a 3-page Patient Care Referral Form or

b. a discharge summary?

2. Does the 3-page referral form include										
a. Completed handwritten demographic data (p. 1)?										
b. Nursing problems and care plan (p. 2)?										
3. Does the discharge summary include										
a. Discharge site										
b. Significant other involved in care										
c. Condition at discharge										
d. Medications										
e. Diet										
f. ADL										
g. Treatments										
h. Teaching										
I. Outpatient follow-up?										

Note. Developed by Nancy Zarle for Beth Israel Hospital, Boston, MA.

APPENDIX B

Quality Assurance Postdischarge Patient Questionnaire

Code: Age:

Reason for hospitalization:

Please check the best answer.

Did nurse explain what to expect when you leave Beth Israel?   Yes _____   No_____

Were the nurse's explanations clear to you?   Yes _____   No _____

Did the nurse answer your questions?   Yes _____   No _____

Did the nurse help you and family/friend to understand what to expect?   Yes _____   No _____

Please answer these questions as clearly as possible. Use the back of this page if necessary.

- How have you felt since leaving the hospital?

- What kind of help have you needed?   Who provides that help?

- What kinds of responsibilities or social activities do you participate in?

- What was the best advice you received from your nurse?

- Has anything unexpected occurred? Please explain.

- What was the most difficult aspect of returning home?

- What advice would you give to another person in your situation?

Please check the column that best describes your current activity best.

	Always	Usually	Sometimes	Never
I feel "good" about myself and my progress.				
I am comfortable enough to go about my usual activities without severe pain				
I know where to get help when I need it.				
I use the help that was recommended by my nurse.				
I am able to meet my spiritual needs satisfactorily.				

Statement				
I visit and do things with other people.				
My home is safe and reasonably well cared for.				
I have adequate clothing.				
I am able to get foods for my diet.				
I eat food recommended for my diet each day.				
I take my medicines according to the doses and times recommended.				
My bowels and bladder work well, without problems.				
I exercise regularly within the recommended limits.				
I am able to feed, bathe, and meet my hygeine needs each day.				
I feel reasonably well rested when I awaken from sleep.				
I am able to follow the doctors' and nurses' suggestions				

Questionnaire completed by: Patient _____ Family member _____ Friend _____

Note. Developed by Celeste Hurley and Nancy Zarle for Beth Israel Hospital, Boston, MA.

Action Plan Worksheet
Part IV: Obstacles and Solutions

Obstacles I May Encounter in This Project	Possible Solutions

* *Note*: The Action Plan Worksheet was adapted from one originally developed by Christine Blaber, MEd; and Kimberly Dash, MPH, Education Development Center Inc., under a grant from the U.S. Department of Education.

Chapter 9

DEFINING THE NURSE'S ROLE IN DISCHARGE PLANNING

LEARNING OBJECTIVES

At the end of this chapter, readers will be able to:

1. Describe different models of nursing involvement and choose the model most appropriate for their setting
2. Establish realistic goals for improving discharge planning at their home institution
3. Define personal career goals and how to improve satisfaction with providing care to the elderly in discharge planning
4. Set an agenda and timetable for future action

Whether or not nurses actually coordinate discharge planning at the hospital, their involvement in the process is essential. Nurses bring special knowledge and skills to the continuing care process. Nurses, however, are only among several professionals who provide their expertise to the discharge planning process. Because no single profession has the knowledge and skill to respond to the many issues faced by patients and their families at hospital discharge, discharge planning lends itself to an interdisciplinary approach (Zarle, 1987; Fitzig, 1988; and Wertheimer & Kleinman, 1990).

In this chapter, the importance of nurses' role in the discharge planning process is examined, along with ways in which that role can be expanded.

MODELS OF NURSING INVOLVEMENT IN DISCHARGE PLANNING

Nurses' input in the discharge planning process is critical whether they are in charge of leading that process or not. The acute care nurse has a number of strengths relevant to the process (Fitzig, 1988). Nurses determine what the patient is able to do and what support services best meet the patient's needs in the basic activities of daily living. They can determine the need for rehabilitation procedures, which may include speech, physical, recreational, or occupational therapy. Nurses can also assess the home for safety and comfort and make appropriate requests for assistive devices as needed: grab bars, elevated toilet seats, flexible shower heads, bath stalls, and walkers. A nurse who is knowledgeable of the community can help patients and their families arrange for services such as transportation, meals-on-wheels programs, and emergency call-button systems.

Preparing for and after discharge, nurses can assist the older patient to get involved in the local senior center for occupational and recreational activities. Acute care nurses can work with public health nurses (or visiting nurses) to do a complete assessment of the patient, home, and community. Public health nurses are able to provide direct care and determine the gaps in services and make referrals.

The following are some basic discharge planning models that focus on personnel employed.

1. *The autonomous discharge planner.* A designated discharge planner has major responsibility for ensuring the patient's continuity of care. (This is usually a nurse who acts as a case finder, consultant, and referral agent.) In this model the discharge planner is relatively autonomous—selecting patients; assessing their needs; and working with family members, hospital staff, and representatives of community agencies to ensure that the patient's posthospital needs are met. In many hospitals, discharge planning is coordinated by social workers because of their familiarity with community services (McNulty, 1988).

2. *Medical and nursing staff working with a discharge planner.* The medical and nursing staffs assume the major responsibility for the patient's continuity of care. Physicians and nurses caring for patients assess their need for posthospital care and then receive follow-up assistance from the discharge planner in arranging for needed ser-

vices. In this way discharge planning is an integral part of the patient care process (McNulty, 1988).

3. *Social workers assisting nurses on specific clinical units.* Social workers who are assigned to specific clinical units work with nurses on the unit to identify the patient's posthospital needs. Discharge planning activities are then divided between them on the basis of the type of care needed (e.g., home care or nursing-home care) (McNulty, 1988).

4. *Medical and nursing staff working with a social worker.* Physicians and nurses assume major responsibility for identifying patients who need posthospital care. They then refer those patients to the social worker, who assumes responsibility for both physical and social needs (e.g., transportation, nursing home referral, consultation with patient and family members). This model resembles the second one where the physician and nurse assume responsibility for the discharge plan, except here they delegate activities to a social worker rather than an official discharge planner (McNulty, 1988).

5. *Collaboration of medical, nursing, social service, and physical therapy staff, in addition to community service providers.* Zarle (1987) argues that early assessment of the patient's need for continuing-care services is what maintains high standards of care. Improvement of the discharge planning process and patient outcome at discharge depends on interdisciplinary collaboration both inside and outside the hospital. (This approach is covered in greater detail in chapter 1.)

6. *An interdisciplinary model of discharge planning coordinated by the hospital's medical staff that involves a clinical pharmacist, floor nurse, community liaison nurse, nutritionist, occupational therapist, physical therapist, psychiatrist, quality assurance and utilization reviewer, social worker, substance abuse counselor, and medical staff (house staff, medical students, and attending physician).* This formally structured model (i.e., having an established protocol for discharge) focuses on identifying functional deficits and acquiring appropriate services both in and out of the hospital to minimize the impact of these problems. Assessment involves five broad areas—cognitive, social, financial, environmental, and access to care—to identify those at risk for problems during hospitalization. Admission assessment and follow-up programs have been identified as two characteristics necessary in a formally structured discharge planning program, for effective care of frail elders (Haddock, 1991).

7.   *A comprehensive discharge planning protocol implemented by a geriatric nurse specialist.* The protocol extends from hospital admission to 2 weeks after discharge. It involves an initial hospital visit, patient assessment, caregiver assessment, interim hospital visits, discharge visits, telephone contact, and telephone outreach after discharge. Research supports the need for comprehensive discharge planning designed for the elderly and implemented by nurse specialists to improve patient outcomes after hospital discharge and to reduce costs. Findings suggest that this model was effective in delaying or preventing rehospitalization of patients who received the protocol (Naylor et al., 1994).

In order to better address the complex in-home care needs of the frail, high-risk patient, increasing numbers of hospitals are developing case management programs to complement their discharge planning efforts. Hospital-based case management is a separate and distinct function from discharge planning. Thus, it requires separate and distinct staff, procedures, and accountability. Discharge planning focuses on episodes of illness related to incidents of acute hospitalization and on the after-care from such incidents. Case management, on the other hand, is a service function directed at coordinating existing resources to assure appropriate and continuous care for individuals on a case-by-case basis. The case manager assumes responsibility for identifying needs, planning and arranging service delivery, and monitoring service provision and outcomes (White, 1986). Unlike discharge planning, case management is ongoing, not just posthospital, and based in the home delivery of personal and medical services. The case manager usually addresses the patient's physical needs for care, counseling needs, assistance with homemaking and other activities of daily living, nutritional needs, legal and financial assistance, transportation, and housing (Clark, 1992). The case manager does not plan patient discharge; the discharge planner is responsible for that. The case manager may be requested to participate in discharge planning if the patient is a client of the case management program. If the case manager is not involved in the discharge planning, proper communication should be in place to enable him or her to become involved after the patient goes home (Simmons & White, 1988). Regardless of which model is followed, comprehensive, structured, and interdisciplinary discharge planning programs that encourage active nursing participation are more likely to be effective. The nurse, though an active participant in discharge planning, cannot do it all. She must rely on the expertise and support provided by other members of the discharge planning team, particularly hospital social workers. Social workers traditionally have been the key link between hospital and community and between the medical, highly technical hospital world and the realities of everyday life (Lawrance, 1988). Social workers are well prepared to assess and deal with many of the psychosocial issues that complicate some cases and often serve as case managers (as can the nurse), linking clients with appropriate community-based resources to address these issues.

IMPLEMENTING PLANS TO IMPROVE DISCHARGE PLANNING: QUESTIONS TO CONSIDER

Now that you have studied discharge planning from the perspectives of all parties, and considered practical, ethical, and procedural issues, you are in a good position to synthesize your knowledge by addressing or readdressing the questions that follow.

1. What are some realistic goals for discharge planning? What are realistic goals for smaller hospitals? For larger hospitals? How might these goals be affected by larger societal, legislative changes? Why are they realistic?

2. How might these goals be accomplished and a reasonable timetable set for completing them?

3. What are your career goals? Can they increase your satisfaction in providing discharge planning to the elderly? What personal strengths do you provide or bring to the planning team? What would you like to improve?

4. What are some of the challenges in developing patients' discharge plans? What strategies are available for responding to these challenges, for example, how do you accomplish your goal without stepping on anyone's toes?

5. Have hospital efforts at cost containment affected discharge planning or staff available to work on discharge plans? What are the ways to improve the process of discharge planning without adding unacceptable costs?

6. What ethical issues have you faced in discharge planning at your institution?

7. How would (or do) you evaluate discharge planning quality issues at work? How would you evaluate the proposed changes to discharge planning that you have suggested in the exercises in this book?

Developing Action Plans to Improve Discharge Planning

Review and revise your action plan. In addition, complete Part V of the action plan to improve discharge planning at your institution. In this part, define the specific action steps related to your objectives and strategies (defined in Part II) and set up a timetable for completing those action steps. See p. 208 for Part V of the action plan.

SUMMARY

The key points of this chapter are:

1. Nurses' input in the discharge planning process is critical whether they control that process or not.
2. Comprehensive, structured, and interdisciplinary discharge planning programs that encourage active nursing participation are more likely to be effective in producing positive discharge outcomes (e.g., delayed or no rehospitalization, greater patient and family satisfaction with the discharge plan, and reduced costs) than less structured, single discipline programs.

REFERENCES

Clark, M. J. (1992). *Nursing in the community*. Norwalk, CT: Appleton & Lange.

Fitzig, C. (1988). Discharge planning: Nursing focus. In P. J. Volland (Ed.), *Discharge planning: An interdisciplinary approach to continuity of care* (pp. 93–117). Owings Mills, MD: National Health Publishing.

Haddock, K. S. (1991). Characteristics of effective discharge planning programs for the frail elderly. *Journal of Gerontological Nursing, 17*(7), 10–14.

Lawrance, F. P. (1988). Discharge planning: Social work focus. In P. J. Volland (Ed.). *Discharge planning: An interdisciplinary approach to continuity of care* (pp. 119–152). Owings Mills, MD: National Health Publishing.

McNulty, E. G. (1988). Discharge planning models. In P. J. Volland (Ed.), *Discharge planning: An interdisciplinary approach to continuity of care* (pp. 21–49). Owings Mills, MD: National Health Publishing.

Naylor, M., Brooten, D., Jones, R., Lavizzo-Mourey, R., Mezey, M., & Pauly, M. (1994). Comprehensive discharge planning for the hospitalized elderly. *Annals of Internal Medicine, 120*, 999–1006.

Simmons, W. J., & White, M. (1988). Case management and discharge planning: Two different worlds. In P. J. Volland (Ed.), *Discharge planning: An interdisciplinary approach to continuity of care* (pp. 217–238). Owings Mills, MD: National Health Publishing.

Wertheimer, D. S., & Kleinman, L. S. (1990). A model for interdisciplinary discharge planning in a university hospital. *The Gerontologist, 30*, 837–840.

White, M. (1986). Case management. In G. L. Maddox (Ed.), *The encyclopedia of aging*. New York: Springer Publishing Co.

Zarle, N. C. (1987). *Continuing care: The process and practice of discharge planning*. Rockville, MD: Aspen Publishers, Inc.

SUGGESTED READINGS

Congdon, J. G. (1990). Managing the incongruities: An analysis of hospital discharge in the elderly. *Communicating Nursing Research, 23*, 11–17.

Reichelt, P. A., & Newcomb, J. (1980). Organizational factors in discharge planning. *Journal of Nursing Administration, 10*, 36–42.

Volland, P. J. (1988). *Discharge planning: An interdisciplinary approach to continuity of care*. Owings Mills, MD: National Health Publishing.

Action Plan Worksheet
Part V: Timeline

Objective #1: _____

_____

_____

Related Strategies: _____

_____

_____

Tasks	J	F	M	A	M	J	J	A	S	O	N	D

* *Note*: The Action Plan Worksheet was adapted from one originally developed by Christine Blaber, MEd, and Kimberly Dash, MPH, Education Development Center, Inc., under a grant from the U.S. Department of Education.

Chapter 10

DEVELOPING DISCHARGE PLANS: A CASE STUDY APPROACH

LEARNING OBJECTIVES

At the end of this chapter, readers will be able to:

1. Conduct a patient, caregiver, and community assessment for an elderly patient prior to discharge to determine that patient's discharge needs
2. Develop a discharge plan that matches the patient with appropriate community resources
3. Evaluate the discharge plan for the case study patient in terms of patient and family satisfaction with the plan
4. Assess and evaluate an institution's discharge planning needs
5. Identify strategies for enlisting administrative support in order to institute necessary changes and improve the quality of discharge planning

Through case studies, nurses practice their skills in assessing elderly patients and in matching elderly patients with appropriate community services. The case study also is a vehicle for institutional assessment. It is a form of evaluation that can help nurses identify the discharge planning needs at their institutions and possible strategies for changing and improving the quality of discharge planning there.

This chapter explains how to create a complete case study. After selecting one of your patients, you will assess and monitor that person's care in the hospital, and plan continuing care services for the patient after his or her discharge.

INTRODUCTION

Provide a brief introductory context for the case by giving (a) the patient's name, (b) name of institution, and (c) members of the discharge planning team. Patient confidentiality should be protected in a case study that may be shared. Do not reveal a patient's real name. You may want to obtain patient permission to participate as a case study. You may also want to protect family, staff and institutional confidentiality.

ASSESSMENT

Assessment entails collecting information about the patient in a variety of ways, including interviews with the patient and significant others, clinical reports and records, and personal observations. Two worksheets for collecting and organizing these data are provided in Appendix B and C of this chapter: the Nursing Assessment Worksheet Guide and a Functional Health Pattern Assessment (FHPA) worksheet. Once data is collected it must be analyzed in order to identify the patient's needs or problems.

Describe briefly when, how, and what data was obtained, and from what source(s). End with a patient problem list. It should include the following:

- general summary of patient status on admission, including anticipated date of discharge
- patient history, including medical history and medications; social, cultural, economic history; source of health care in the community; significant others; functional and physical assessment data
- source(s) of information
- FHPA pattern areas, briefly described with deviations from expected norms noted

- problems identified from assessment data, and how you determined they were problems
- anticipated discharge status

PLANNING

Develop a plan to address the patient's short- and long-term needs. First, set priorities and decide which problems are nursing problems and which ones should be dealt with by other people (e.g., patient, family members and significant others, other primary continuing care team members, the collaborative primary care team). Next, develop a nursing care plan, detailing expected outcomes and procedures for addressing each problem. A Nursing Care Plan form (Appendix D) is provided to help organize this information, along with a decision-making model (Appendix E) to help match the patient with skilled and supportive services in the community. The decision-making model outlines, factors, that put patients at increased risk for poor postdischarge outcomes and provides appropriate action steps that nurses can take to reduce the likelihood of poor outcomes and improve continuing care for patients.

A case study should mention how decisions were made and who participated. The planning section should discuss setting priorities, assigning responsibility for each problem, and developing and documenting the nursing care plan (diagnosis; expected short- and long-term outcomes; and nursing plan, including nursing orders).

IMPLEMENTATION

Setting a plan in motion to meet the patient's needs after discharge from the acute care setting entails intellectual, interpersonal, and technical skills, as well as decision making, observation, and communication. The nurse must implement both a nursing care plan and a medical care plan, although it may be possible to integrate these.

In pursuing the implementation phase of the case study, consider content, method(s) of delivery, and person(s) with whom you communicate. A discharge summary guideline form is provided in Appendix F of this chapter to help organize information. Discuss any of the following questions that are relevant:

1. What instructions were communicated, and to whom, to help the patient adhere to the medical plan?
2. Did the patient require any nursing information as a result of the medical plan in order to avoid new complications or problems? If so, how was this conveyed and to whom?
3. Was any instruction given to the patient, the family and/or significant others to clarify why the patient should or should not do certain things? If so, how was this done?
4. If continuing care providers were contacted, who were they, how did communication take place, and what was the reason for the communication?
5. How were the nursing orders, their results, and the patient's response to them recorded? To whom were written records conveyed?

EVALUATION

Because the major concern is making sure that the patient's needs are met, you need mechanisms to learn from patients and their families whether the care and services provided were satisfactory and delivered in a timely, efficient, and effective manner. You can also obtain information from continuing care providers in the community. Obtaining this feedback makes it possible not only to improve the discharge planning process for other patients with similar needs, but also to ensure that the patient's ongoing and perhaps changing needs are being met.

Evaluation is an ongoing process that occurs each time a nurse updates the nursing care plan. Initial conclusions provide the basis for setting goals, anticipating outcomes, and making decisions; therefore, it is necessary to see if achieved outcomes coincide with expected outcomes, or if changes are necessary.

Various methods of evaluation are used in nursing; the key to effective evaluation is making sure that the method utilized is tailored to the goals being evaluated. In other words, nurses should generate a list of process and outcome objectives they would like to achieve regarding the patient in their case study. For example, process objectives might include involving the patient and the family in planning continuing care after discharge from the hospital and patient and family education about medical regimen after discharge. The outcomes might include patient and family satisfaction with the discharge and continuing care plan, greater patient adherence to the post-discharge medical regimen, and no readmission within 12 months of discharge.

In preparing a case study, you may include a Postdischarge Patient Questionnaire, Continuing Care Documentation Audit Criteria form, and a Primary Nurse Questionnaire, in your evaluation; copies of the first two forms are included in chapter 8 and the latter is provided in Appendix F of this chapter. The evaluation report should concentrate on the following questions:

1. What evaluation activities did you conduct? When?
2. How were they documented?
3. What types of information were you recording (e.g., services offered and provided, patient's responses, efforts to address both immediate and long-term care needs, follow-up procedures)?
4. What did you learn?

CONCLUSION

Your conclusion should describe both observations and recommendations based on what you have learned.

Include remarks not only about the individual patient, but also concerning your assessment and evaluation of your institution's discharge planning needs. Identify strategies for enlisting administrative support in order to institute necessary changes and improve the quality of discharge planning. Is there anything you would do differently next time? If yes, what?

APPENDIX A

Sample Case Study*

Introduction

Background.   Mrs. Esther Carmichael is a 74-year-old widow who was admitted to Springfield Hospital with severe, unremitting diarrhea. Her diarrhea had been present over the past several years but was in remission for a short period of time during which Mrs. Carmichael lived at a nursing home. When Mrs. Carmichael was discharged from the nursing home to her apartment, she began to experience diarrhea again, a condition usually aggravated by food. These symptoms persisted for 2 to 3 months prior to admission. Mrs. Carmichael suffered from diarrhea throughout the night and her symptoms were not relieved by her usual medicines (Questran® and Azulfidine®). Last year, Mrs. Carmichael underwent a proctoscopy and the gastroenterologist noted an area of friability and edema in her colon. A more recent proctoscopy revealed indications of ulcerative colitis. As a result, Mrs. Carmichael was placed on prednisone 40 mg per day and vitamins. However, her diarrhea persisted and she was eventually admitted to the hospital for total parenteral nutrition and no solid foods.

Status on admission.   Mrs. Carmichael was very weak and dehydrated on admission. She weighed 77 pounds and stood 5 feet, 1 inch tall. Her lungs had some inspiratory bronchi; her heart rhythm was regular and rapid at 110 beats per minute. Her skin was dry and hung wasted on her body. She had plus 2 edema of her lower extremities, and extremities were very tender to the touch. Her pedal pulses were absent and her reflexes hypoactive. She also complained of burning and marked discomfort in her legs. Her blood pressure was 160/90 and she had a temperature of 99° F. Mrs. Carmichael was totally alert and oriented to time and place and knew why she was in the hospital. She reported being allergic to penicillin, codeine, and morphine. She was strong enough to use a commode at her bedside with some assistance.

---

* This case was adapted from one originally developed by Elizabeth Thoms, RN, BSN, a participant in the pilot version of the discharge planning educational program at the Beth Israel Hospital in Boston, Massachusetts.

The following are the results of lab tests administered at admission:

albumin: 3.1
serum sodium: 128
carbon dioxide: 32
potassium: 2.6
osmolality serum: 263
red blood cells: 3.23
hemoglobin: 9.1
hematocrit: 28.1

Functional Health Pattern Assessment

Medical history. Mrs. Carmichael's past medical history includes:

1987 Pulmonary fibrosis, which did not appear in a chest x-ray in 1984, thought to have been caused by Dilantin therapy
1987 Inflammatory bowel disease
1979 Esophageal myotomy for symptoms of dysphasia and regurgitation of food related to diverticulum
1977 Cancer removed from lower left eyelid
1966 Seizure disorder secondary to a head injury from a fall
1960 Cholecystectomy
1958 Total hysterectomy
1949 Appendectomy

Medications include the following:

- Mysoline® at 50 mg, two pills 3 times a day
- Elavil® at 50 to 75 mg at bedtime
- Azulfidine® at 1 gram every 8 hours
- Lactose-free diet
- Questran® once per day

Health perception and health management. Mrs. Carmichael said that she is discouraged and tired. She has been living in an elderly housing complex for the past 8 years; for the last 4 years she has been living alone. A VNA nurse sees her once per month. Mrs. Carmichael stated that she can care for herself and has not had any major problems until the past couple of months when her diarrhea became worse and she did not dare leave her apartment. On admission she said that she was having up to 25 bowel movements per day. Mrs. Carmichael had lived in a nursing home for 6 months in 1988 because of her diarrhea, and she said that she was proud of the fact that she was able to return home and care for herself.

Because of the pulmonary fibrosis, Mrs. Carmichael must limit her activity and take breaks between activities. Mrs. Carmichael has chronic advantageous sounds in both of her lung bases. Her stools are brown and watery without any signs of blood.

Mrs. Carmichael does not smoke and never has. She also does not drink alcohol. She has been taking Elavil since her husband's death in 1985. Her health care providers are Dr. Haley and Raymond VNA. Discharge is anticipated after home hyperal therapy is evaluated and bowel movements occur at a reasonable number per day.

Self-perception and self-concept.   Mrs. Carmichael feels that she has had her share of illness and is depressed because she is unable to do many of the social activities that she has enjoyed in the past. She feels self-conscious about her weight loss and needs to purchase clothes that fit her. Lately, she has been bothered by abdominal cramps that accompany her diarrhea and has been taking Demerol® by mouth, *pro re nata*. She does not want to be a burden to her three sons, two of whom live in the area. She hopes that she will improve while hospitalized so that she can return to her apartment. She would also like to participate in the senior citizen activities that she has always enjoyed in the past.

Roles and relationships.   Mrs. Carmichael lives alone and has done so for 4 years with one 6-month stay in February, 1988, in a nursing home after her last hospitalization. Two of her three sons, Steve and Ben, live within a 20-mile radius of her. One son buys Mrs. Carmichael's groceries and checks in on her weekly; he is also the executor of her will. Mrs. Carmichael's third son, Jeff, has a new family and calls on her when he can. She is concerned that Jeff will have her put on life-support systems when she becomes critically ill and does not want to have her life prolonged in that manner. Jeff had a very difficult time with his father's death. He insisted that his father be placed on a respirator prior to the father's death.

Mrs. Carmichael was a homemaker all her life and cared for her invalid husband 10 years before his death in 1985 of a severe stroke. Mrs. Carmichael is not currently covered by Medicaid but has been in the past.

Coping and stress. Mrs. Carmichael states that she takes one day at a time. She has been taking Elavil at night since her husband's death to help her sleep. She states that she has been depressed since her diarrhea has increased. This has left her unable to socialize outside her apartment. She laments that she is unable to visit her son Jeff in Ohio. She enjoys crocheting and watches game shows on television in the evening.

Cognitive and perceptual. Mrs. Carmichael scored a 28—a near perfect score—on the Folstein Mini Mental State Exam. She is knowledgeable about her low residue, lactose-free diet, and her medications. She understands when to take her medications. She wears bifocals and hears well. She asks physicians about her treatments, and all her questions are appropriate. She wants all of her caretakers to call her Esther and she remembers everyone's name.

Activity and exercise. Mrs. Carmichael is unable to walk more than a few yards without resting because of her chronic lung condition. When her diarrhea is frequent and she is experiencing cramps, she stays in bed and uses a bedside commode at the hospital. At home she has been able to make it to her bathroom. Other than the commode, she does not need the use of any assistive devices.

Nutrition and metabolic. Mrs. Carmichael is on a low-residue, lactose-free diet. Her son does her grocery shopping. She reports an excellent appetite but states that eating food has increased her diarrhea. She also states that in the past month she has been "cheating" on her lactose-free diet because she is always "starving and craving ice cream and cheese." She says that eating these foods has aggravated her condition even more. Esther is now only 89% of her ideal body weight. She was 50 pounds heavier before onset of her ulcerative colitis. Her skin is also very dry and her perianal area is sore from the loose stools.

Elimination. Lately she has been experiencing up to 25 loose, watery, brown, guaic negative stools per day. She states that she does not have any bladder problems and her urinalysis is normal.

Sleep and rest. Mrs. Carmichael states that her diarrhea decreases during the night because she is not eating. However she continues to have bowel movements every few hours and she naps in between. Lately, she has felt tired all day long because the pain in her swollen legs also keeps her up at night.

Values and beliefs. Mrs. Carmichael is a Protestant but has been unable to attend church this past year. She is visited by the minister of her church fairly regularly. She believes that there is life after death and that she will be reunited with her husband in heaven. She has expressed interest in having a living will so that her sons will know her wishes when her "time comes."

Sexuality and reproductive. Mrs. Carmichael has had four pregnancies. Her oldest child died in infancy and she has three living sons. She had a hysterectomy when she was in her forties because of fibroid cysts. She does not have a significant other at this time and is not sexually active.

Anticipated discharge status. The discharge goal for Mrs. Carmichael is to have her return home on nighttime hyperalimentation infusions with assistance of a total parenteral nutrition (TPN) home health care agency and VNA visits. Mrs. Carmichael will not ingest food by eating except for vital supplements to avoid diarrhea.

Planning Patient Hospital Care and Continuing Care

Patient problems. Mrs. Carmichael's primary problem was her nutritional status. She was starved and dehydrated on admission, and this condition had to be addressed before any other long-term goals could be attained. After nursing staff initiated hyper-alimentation (hyperal) therapy, Mrs. Carmichael's nutritional status improved and she was able to participate in her discharge planning.

Mrs. Carmichael's comfort level also required immediate nursing attention. She was suffering from abdominal cramps and leg pain due to her edema. With intravenous Lasix®, Mrs. Carmichael's edema subsided and she was started on Lasix® 3 times per week.

Nursing staff monitored Mrs. Carmichael's nutritional status daily, including her electrolytes. Hyperal was prescribed daily. Mrs.

Carmichael also received several units of packed cells, which helped revitalize her. With her TPN status, frequency of bowel movements lessened as did her cramps. She was then placed on Hycodan® syrup, which helped reduce abdominal cramping.

Patient Care Plan

Nursing diagnoses	Expected outcomes	Nursing order
Alteration in bowel elimination: ulcerative colitis, 20–25 stools/day.	Patient's number of stools will decrease to a manageable number per day prior to discharge from the hospital.	NPO status. Commode at bedside. Keep stool chart. Imodium every 6 hours.
Alteration in nutrition less than body requirements. Admission weight = 77 pounds.	Patient will have her nutrition requirements met with nighttime hyperalimentation infusion and vital supplements and will show an improvement in nutrition status and weight gain prior to hospital discharge.	Daily weight. Monitor lab values daily and report changes to MD. Encourage vital supplements. Assess lungs every 4 hrs and report adventitious sounds to MD. Assess patient for peripheral edema daily. Change Hickmann dressing Tuesday and Friday. Assess for signs and symptoms of infection of insertion site. Vitals every 4 hours. pH and specific gravity every 8 hours.

Patient Care Plan (cont.)

Nursing diagnoses	Expected outcomes	Nursing order
Self-care deficit: nighttime hyperal. Note that the patient will have hyperal bags delivered pre-spiked with lines primed. She will only be expected to attach herself and detach in the PM and AM and to flush the Hickmann each time this is done. All other responsibilities lie with the TPN nurse and the VNA nurse.	Patient will be able to hook herself up and detach herself from hyperal every PM and AM and repeat demonstration of procedures to RN prior to discharge, and perform procedure 4 nights prior to discharge, every night.	Demonstrate proper attachment and detachment of hyperal to patient using TPN guidelines and techniques. Teach patient signs and symptoms of infection. Teach patient urine testing. Teach patient to trouble shoot infusion pump. Teach patient sterile technique when attaching and detaching hyperal. Teach patient how to clamp the catheter. Teach patient infusion rate and when to decrease infusion rate prior to detachment. Review complications associated with central venous catheters (TPN manual).
Alternation in comfort: intestinal cramping.	Patient's cramps will decrease with TPN and will be	Assess patient's comfort level *pro re nata*, use pain

Patient Care Plan (cont.)

Nursing diagnoses	Expected outcomes	Nursing order
	controlled with Hycodan syrup every 4–6 hours.	scale 1–10. Ask patient to name her level of comfort and record. Assess efficacy of pain medications 30–45 minutes after administration. Maintain TPN except for vital supplements. Encourage mouth care. Offer diversional activities.
Discharge planning	Patient will have needs met at home with the help of: • VNA daily visits • TPN biweekly visit • Homemaker daily visit • Emergency button system • Meals on Wheels when the patient is ready to eat again • Bedside commode	Arrange patient care conference with all disciplines involved including TPN nurse, VNA nurse, MD, primary RN, dietary, and social worker. Expected Discharge: 3/17/89

Care Plan Implementation

Once stable on hyperal, Mrs. Carmichael's primary nurse organized a patient care conference, which included Mrs. Carmichael; her two physicians, including the gastroenterologist; her primary nurse; a social worker; the TPN nurse from the home care company providing hyperal services; the VNA nurse who would be assisting Mrs. Carmichael at home (and who had assisted her in the past); a dietitian; and Mrs. Carmichael's son, Steve. In the meeting, participants discussed whether Mrs. Carmichael had the cognitive and physical ability to assist herself at home with nighttime infusions of hyperal. The TPN nurse had made three teaching and assessing visits to Mrs. Carmichael prior to the care conference and felt that Mrs. Carmichael showed good potential for home hyperal infusions. Her main concern was that Esther might "wear herself out" trying to care for herself and her hyperal as well. Participants decided, therefore, that the TPN company would spike and prime each hyperal bag and store three bags in the refrigerator so that all Esther would need to do would be to flush her line and attach her hyperal to her Hickmann catheter. Afterward, the VNA nurse would be available daily to assess Mrs. Carmichael's progress and the TPN nurse would assist Esther with the first week of home infusions, being on call for problems or questions. Care conference participants decided that a bedside commode would be necessary for the nighttime so that Mrs. Carmichael would not need to walk with the infusion pump to the bathroom. Esther would have a homemaker stop in daily and meals-on-wheels when or if she was able to resume food. Daily, and if necessary twice a day, visits from the visiting nurse were anticipated. Steve would check in on her weekly and help her with bills, groceries, and errands.

Although Esther understood her medication regimen and was able to take her medications without any problems prior to admission, her physician would streamline Mrs. Carmichael's medications, sending her home with only the absolutely necessary medications. The physician also suggested that two of Mrs. Carmichael's closest friends, who also live in the same building, could learn some of the basic hyperal infusion tasks in case Esther needed some support. An emergency button service was also ordered for Mrs. Carmichael and will be installed prior to her discharge. Mrs. Carmichael has also applied for Medicaid with the help of the social worker and she should be accepted as she has been on Medicaid in the past.

Mrs. Carmichael had daily visits from the TPN nurse with instruction on her hyperal infusion. The nurse taught Mrs. Carmichael to use the infusion pump and to trouble shoot for malfunctions in the system. Mrs. Carmichael also learned the signs and symptoms of infection and was able to repeat these back to the TPN nurse. For four nights prior to discharge, Mrs. Carmichael was able to flush her line and hook herself up to her hyperal nightly. The nurse provided Mrs. Carmichael with a list of phone numbers to call if she experiences problems. In addition, the TPN nurse showed Mrs. Carmichael how to use her emergency button service unit.

Prior to hospital discharge, Mrs. Carmichael experienced fewer bowel movements and minimal discomfort. Her edema was gone and her lab values were returning to normal. Her weight increased to 84 pounds from the 77 at admission. She was able to walk independently with less pain in her legs and reported feeling stronger. She stated that she felt good about going home and felt competent to administer her nighttime hyperal. She was relieved that she would have a strong support system at home.

Evaluation of the Continuing Care Plan

Using the Beth Israel Hospital's Postdischarge Patient Questionnaire, Mrs. Carmichael was questioned 3 months after discharge about the quality of her discharge plan and her satisfaction with it. Information regarding services offered and provided, patient's perceived physical and social well-being, and ability to follow medical regimen were documented. Mrs. Carmichael responded that she felt better since leaving the hospital. Resuming some of her social activities, like Bingo twice per week, cheered her up. She also noted that she has learned to be positive and remain calm about her medical regimen even though she finds infusing the hyperal to be difficult. Most important, she noted that nothing unexpected has occurred. However, she still reported some problems with her bowels, stating that they work well without problems only "sometimes."

Conclusion

Overall, Mrs. Carmichael's case was a successful one and proved that by working with a multidisciplinary discharge planning team, the nurse could help ensure that the discharge plan was more accurately suited to the patient's continuing care needs. The most prominent gap in discharge planning at Springfield Hospital was the absence of follow-up evaluation instruments to document the quality of the discharge plan and patient satisfaction with that plan. Mrs. Carmichael's primary nurse has been instrumental in educating nursing administration about this lack of instrumentation. As a result, administrators are taking steps to adapt and revise evaluation instruments used by other hospitals in the region, including the Beth Israel Hospital instruments employed in this case study.

APPENDIX B

Beth Israel Hospital Nursing Services: Nursing Assessment Worksheet Guide

Introductory Statement

I would like to ask you a few questions about yourself and your usual daily activities at home to help us make your care as individual as possible while you are here in the hospital.

Reason for Hospitalization

What health problem led you to come to the hospital at this time?
How long have you had this problem?
What do you know about your illness?
What are your expectations of this hospitalization?
What things worry you at this time?

Other Medical Problems

Have you ever been hospitalized before?
If yes, for what purpose?
Do you have any medical problems besides the problem for which you
    are being admitted?

Social, Cultural, Economic History

Do you live in your own home? An apartment?
How many stairs must you climb?
What is your occupation? Are you retired?
What was the date of your last employment?
Has your illness affected your family or your usual way of life?
What is your ethnic background?
Do you have any religious practicies you would like us to honor?
Will the cost of this hospitalization cause any problems for you
    financially?

Significant Others

Who do you live with?

Tell me about the members of your family (friends).

Will anyone at home need assistance while you are in the hospital?

While you are in the hospital, do you expect to have anyone visit you? If yes, who?

Do you have someone able to care for you when you are discharged, if you should need help?

Medications Taken Prior to Admission

Have you been taking medication or treatments before your admission to the hospital?

If yes, what is the drug or treatment, the dosage, the usual times you take them?

Can you explain the purpose of the drugs (treatment).

What medicines do you take that can be purchased over the counter?

Allergies

Are there any drugs or foods that you cannot use?

If yes, what is the drug or food?

What happens when you take them?

Functional Data on Admission

Food habits

Do you have any restrictions on your diet; for example are you diabetic or do you have to follow a low-sodium diet because of your high blood pressure?

Tell me about your eating habits at home; for example, do you eat all three meals, skip breakfast, have a big lunch?

Tell me exactly what you ate the day before you came into the hospital.

Level of activity

Are you able to get around the house, do errands, and take care of your personal needs independently, or do you need assistance?

If you need help, explain what you need.

Personal hygiene

Tell me about your usual routine for daily hygiene.
Do you prefer a bath or a shower? When? How often?
Do you need assistance in grooming?
What do you do for mouth care, denture care?
Do you have any special soaps, lotions, or other items that you may
need here?

Elimination

We will be checking to make sure that your voiding and elimination
patterns remain as close to normal as possible while you are hospitalized, so we would like to know your usual pattern; for example,
do you have any problem passing your urine or stool?
Do you have daily bowel movement?
Do you use a laxative?
If yes, what kind and how often?

Female reproductive status

What was the date of your last menstrual period?
When do you expect your next period?
Have you used, or are you using any particular method of birth
control?
Do you have any menstrual problems?
Any postmenopausal problems?
When was the date of your last PAP smear?
Do you examine your own breasts?
If yes, how often?

Recreation and hobbies

What do you normally do for recreation or to pass time?
Tell me about your special intersts or hobbies.

Other

Do you smoke?
If yes, what do you smoke?
If cigarettes, how many packs a day?

Do you partake of alcoholic beverages?
If yes, what kind? How often?
Can you tell me of any special requests that you would like us to honor while you are here?

Physical Assessment Data

Patient status on admission

Subjective data from patient of family:
Height:
Weight:
Temperature:
General Appearance:

Vision

Incxlude use of prosthesis, descriptors and information, if appropriate: inflammation, date of last eye exam, use of medication, discharge, or muscular control.

Ears

Include voice and tone needed for patient to distinguish sound (low, moderate, loud).
Include whether hearing is partial or complete and whether the patient is able to lip-read.
Include whether patient wears a hearing-aid.

Mouth

Indicate if patient has teeth/dentures.
Describe condition of teeth.
Include color, turgor, and intactness of mucous membranes.
Include any unusual speech pattern, such as lisping, stutter, or use of esophageal speech.
Include patient's ability to chew and swallow.
Also include date of last dental exam.
Indicate the presence of lip sores and breath smell.

Neuro/mental status

Include use of consciousness (i.e., alert and quick to respond to stimuli, drowsy, semiconscious, or dfficult to arouse).

Orientation—to time, place, and person. May also include ability to recall past or present events.

Include pupillary status (i.e., pupils equal, round, and reactive to light).

Emotional expression—appropriateness of behavior and affect.

Spontaneous speech.

Comprehension.

Skin

Include cleanliness, presence of unusual discoloration, pallor, rubor cyanosis, and jaundice.

Include whether broken, intact, any sensitivity to heat or cold.

May include the following descriptors: rashes, decubitis, itching, lesions, pigmentation.

Include descriptors about hair: color, texture, cleaniness, distribution.

Include information about nails: color, length, cleanliness.

Include other abnormalities; for example, indicate presence, location, and degree of edema.

Respiratory

Include rate changes, depth, rhythm, (regular, or irregular, such as Cheyne Stokes).

Indicate whether the chest is clear or abnormal.

Dyspnea—include any use of the accessory respiratory muscles and the presence of sounds, such as stridor or wheezes.

Respiratory aids—include type, such as medihalers and any abnormal respiratory opening, such as a tracheostomy.

Cardiovascular

Pulse—record pulse obtained, indicating if regular or irregular. Indicate site pulse was obtained by checking the appropriate space (apical or radial).

Irregular, describe.

Blood pressure—minimum requirement, blood pressure in both arms lying, sitting, or standing; indicate the position selected.

Record postural signs if patient has a complaint of dizziness of another symptom that would warrant this.

Peripheral pulses—obtain if indicated, and record the absence or presence.

Mobility

May include whether patient ambulates with assistance, a supportive aid, such as a person, crutches, braces, etc.

Include the location and level of extremity loss and type of prosthesis, if indicated.

Describe whether movement is coordinated, uncoordinated, convulsive spastic, or tremorous.

Describe any deformities, such as contractures.

Describe gait (i.e., coordination and balance).

Appliance (self-explanatory).

Nursing Problems and Plan

Use the space provided to work out the nursing problem identified from the assessment data and the corresponding care.

Anticipated Discharge Date

Include a general time frame and the place to which patient is expected to return.

Source. Beth Israel Hospital, Boston, MA

APPENDIX C: BETH ISRAEL HOSPITAL NURSING SERVICES

Functional Health Pattern Assessment (FHPA)— Admission Assessment Criteria

General Summary

Level of consciousness
Allergies

Time of admission
Admitted from
Vital signs, height, weight
Persons accompanying patient
Pertinent clinical data
Valuables, glasses, dentures, prosthesis

Pattern Areas

Health perception–health management

General health (PMH and PSH)
Smoking, ETOH
Reason for admission
Medications
Health care provider

Self-perception–self-concept

Perception of illness
Expectations of hospitalization
Impact of illness on self/others

Roles–relationships

Name of person to be notified in case of an emergency
Living situation/support system
Occupation

Coping–stress

Major stresses
Usual coping mechanism

Cognitive–perceptual

Prosthesis and disposition
Language spoken
Sensory perceptions (pain, vision)
Level of orientation
Name wishes to be called by

Activity–exercise

Exercise pattern
Assistive devices

Nutrition–metabolic

Diet
Weight loss/gain
Skin status

Elimination

Bowel and bladder patterns

Sleep–rest

Sleep patterns

Values–beliefs

Religious practice/needs

Sexuality–reproductive

Pertinent pattern information

Anticipated Discharge Status

Assessment

Plan

Source. Beth Israel Hospital, Boston, MA

APPENDIX D: NURSING CARE PLAN

Nursing history   Formulated by _____   Date ____

Nursing diagnosis	Expected outcome	Nursing care plan with nursing orders

APPENDIX E: CONTINUING CARE PLANNING DECISION MATRIX

High-risk DRGs	High-risk patients	Placement of risks	Educational risks
1. Usually associated with placement or intensive "after" acute needs	1. Variant within DRG**	1. Any length-of-stay increase due to a lack of services/ resources	1. Intensive patient educational needs
2. LOS* rather than DRG** frame increases	2. Patient History	2. Highly unusual resource needs	2. Family education
3. Difficult clinical management			3. High readmits

Actions

High-risk DRGs	High-risk patients	Placement of risks	Educational risks
1. Preadmission policy	1. Generic screening	1. Analyze patterns	1. QA†† on readmissions
2. Integrated involvement: community resources	2. UR† and RN case finding	2. Cultivate resources	2. Heighten teaching/ patient education awareness
3. Staff education	3. If needed, strengthen social services	3. Attend meetings	3. Decrease patient dependence
	4. Staff education		

Notes. * Length of stay.
 ** Diagnostic related groups.
 † Utilization review.
 †† Quality assurance.

Source. Beth Israel Hospital, Boston, MA

APPENDIX F: DISCHARGE SUMMARY GUIDELINES

By the time of the discharge, the primary nurse will ensure that a discharge summary is documented in the patient's record.

Criteria

1. There will be a discharge summary title.
2. The date and time of the discharge will be recorded.
3. Documentation will indicate the patient's significant other's knowledge about each of the following:

• Discharge site	Where is the patient being discharged?
• Significant other involved in care	Who is available to assist patient with hospital care?
• Condition at discharge—physical and emotional	What is significant about the patient's physical and emotional status?
• Medications	Has the patient been instructed about name, dosage, schedule of administration, action, and side effects?
• Diet	On what type of diet is the patient being discharged? Has the patient received necessary instruction about food selection, buying, and preparation? What is the patient's response to dietary limitation?
• ADL	Will the patient be able to resume normal activities of bathing, eating, dressing, etc., without assistance? If assistance is needed, how will those needs be met? Special devices, etc.?
• Special teaching or treatment	Does the patient have special needs and treatments that will be continued upon discharge (colostomy care, dressing changes)?

| | Has the patient or s. o. been properly instructed? Discuss specifics of treatment plan that are significant for follow-up. |
| • Follow-up plans | Who will provide follow-up care (physician, clinic, nurse)? What plans have been made for the next appointment? |

4. Additional information is noted if necessary.

_____ RN

Note. From *Continuing care: The process and practice of discharge planning* (p. 57) by N. C. Zarle, 1987. Rockville, MD: Aspen. Copyright 1987 by Aspen Publishers, Inc. Reprinted with permission.

INDEX

S *Springer Publishing Company*

GERONTOLOGY REVIEW GUIDE FOR NURSES

Elizabeth Chapman Shaid, RN, MSN, CRNP
Kay Huber, DEd, RN, CRNP

This book distills key concepts of gerontology and older adult care into a rapidly accessible format. Its multiple purposes include ANA certification exams review, continuing education, basic nursing education, curriculum development. It also serves as a tool for developing standards of care and critical pathways for care delivery, or just as a quick reference. The twenty-three chapters cover everything from the most prominent theories in aging to physical changes and psychosocial considerations in aging. An appendix provides useful tips for test taking.

Partial Contents:

Overview of the Field
 • Gerontological Nursing Practice
 • Demographics of Aging
 • Aging Definitions and Theories

Age-Related Physical Changes and Common Problems
 • Cardiovascular System
 • Gastrointestinal System
 • Sensory System
 • Musculoskeletal System
 • Human Sexuality and the Aging Process
 • Medications

Psychosocial and Health Maintenance Issues
 • Cognition and Mental Health
 • Managing Behavioral Problems
 • Falls

Nursing and Health Care Management
 • Nursing/Health Assessment
 • The Organization of Health Care Services for the Elderly
 • Ethical and Legal Considerations and Issues

1996   244pp   0-8261-9120-7   softcover

536 Broadway, New York, NY 10012-3955 • (212) 431-4370 • Fax (212) 941-7842

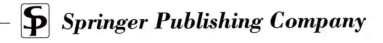 *Springer Publishing Company*

STRENGTHENING GERIATRIC NURSING EDUCATION

Terry Fulmer, RN, PhD, FAAN and
Marianne Matzo, PhD, RN, CS, Editors

This book is designed to promote geriatric content in the basic nursing curriculum, in order to make sure new nurse graduates are properly prepared to care for the growing numbers of elderly in the United States. Distinguished nurse educators review the current state of geriatrics and gerontology in the nursing curriculum, and make recommendations for fully incorporating them into the program of study.

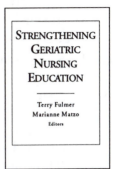

Partial Contents:

- Why Good Ideas Have Not Gone Far Enough: The State of Geriatric Nursing Education, *Mathy Mezey*
- Barriers in Nursing Education, *Marianne Matzo*
- Incorporating Geriatrics into the Licensure and Accreditation Process, *Terry Fulmer* and *Mary Tellis Nyack*
- Expanding Clinical Experiences, *May L. Wykle* and *Carol M. Musil*
- Student Resistance: Overcoming Ageism, *Carla Mariano*
- Normal Aging and Physiology, *Mary (Mickie) Burke* and *Susan E. Sherman*
- Psychiatric Mental Health, *Carol M. Musil and May L. Wykle*
- Elimination and Skin Problems, *Marie O'Toole*

1995   200pp   0-8261-8940-7   hardcover

536 Broadway, New York, NY 10012-3955 • (212) 431-4370 • Fax (212) 941-7842